I0552604

SURVIVING SHIT CREEK

ONE NURSE'S STORY OF BREAKDOWNS, BREAKTHROUGHS, AND TRANSFORMATION

Lori Ann Lewicki, MSN, RN, CCRN, PHRN

Aurora Corialis Publishing

Pittsburgh, PA

SURVIVING SHIT CREEK: ONE NURSE'S STORY OF BREAKDOWNS, BREAKTHROUGHS, AND TRANSFORMATION

Copyright © 2024 by Lori Ann Lewicki

All rights reserved. No part of this book may be used, reproduced, stored in a retrieval system, or transmitted by any means—electronic, mechanical, photocopy, microfilm, recording, or otherwise—without written permission from the publisher, except in the case of brief quotations embodied in critical articles or reviews. For more information, address: cori@auroracorialispublishing.com.

All external reference links utilized in this book have been validated to the best of our ability and are current as of publication.

The publisher and the author make no guarantees concerning the level of success you may experience by following the advice and strategies contained in this book, and the reader accepts the risk that results will differ for each individual.

Neither the author nor the publisher assumes any responsibility for errors, omissions, or contrary interpretations of the subject matter herein. Any perceived slight of an individual or organization is purely unintentional.

To ensure privacy and confidentiality, some names or other identifying characteristics of the persons included in this book may have been changed. All the personal examples of the author's own life and experiences have not been altered.

Printed in the United States of America

Edited by: Allison Hrip, Aurora Corialis Publishing

Cover Design: Karen Captline, BetterBe Creative

Paperback ISBN: 978-1-958481-32-5

Ebook ISBN: 978-1-958481-33-2

Praise for Surviving Shit Creek

"Life can be unpleasantly complex, but there is always hope. I love that Lori Ann Lewicki wrote *Surviving Shit Creek* in such an authentic way, showing us that you really can get through the storms and come out on the other side of the rainbow. As someone who has also been through her fair share of trials, I appreciate how she shared all her emotions along the way and challenges the reader to change their thinking with incremental shifts to better their lives. We all deserve to be happy, and I think that's the biggest takeaway. This is a great book, especially for those in healthcare, to make sure they are taking care of themselves so they can then also support the people who need them most."

Jennifer Silbaugh
Author of *A Dove in the Shadows: My Mental Health Recovery Journey from Patient to Professional*

"Lori Ann Lewicki clearly has a passion for helping nurses love themselves and fall back in love with their jobs. The transparency and vulnerability shared in her book forced me to look inside and become more self-aware of my own thoughts and feelings, even the ones that at times feel uncomfortable. Growing through challenges is a lesson everyone will have to eventually learn, and Lori's book will help you through the process by seeing firsthand what it looks like to find the lesson in anger, frustration, and dark emotions, knowing that those feelings won't last forever. This book is a must read for anyone wanting to rediscover the power and passion within themselves!"

Desiree Petrich
Founder of Intentional Action, LLC | Author of *Taking Intentional Action: How to Choose the Life You Lead*

Disclaimer

This book is not designed to give medical advice. It is not intended to be an all-knowing guide. I am just one nurse telling my story of overcoming. I am here to be a beacon of hope to others.

There needs to be a trigger warning for this book. I am blunt, and sometimes too honest, but I promise to never sugarcoat shit. I don't do it in my personal *or* professional life. When someone asks my opinion I ask back, "Do you want me to tell you the truth or lie to you?" I give you the option to have the sugarcoated bullshit answer, but at least I warn you that's exactly what you are getting.

So if you have had serious trauma, sexual assault, or abuse (that you have not dealt with yet), you may not want to read this. This book is how I dealt with all the shit life has thrown at me. I am not perfect, nor do I claim to be. This is my life from my perspective and my opinion. If you can't handle those, then please move along.

If you have trauma, I hope you will be inspired to heal it or use the techniques I share in this book to help you enjoy nursing again like you did when you first graduated and were filled with the wonderment of helping others. I do not claim to be an expert. I am not the end-all-be-all for coaching. I am just one nurse telling her story in hopes of inspiring others.

I am a female. I write from a female perspective, using the pronouns she/hers. I mean no malice by only using female pronouns in this book. I do not mean to offend any male nurse or imply that you are not important. Male nurses are very valuable to the profession, and I love working with them. It especially makes lifting and turning patients so much easier. My friend always teases me at work that I only ask for his help when I need to lift a patient. (That comment is for my favorite nurse to work with, and I am not mentioning his name so I don't have to pay him royalties.) In all seriousness though, we need both males and females as nurses. We each bring unique gifts to the profession.

Dedication

The font in this book is used specifically for those who are dyslexic to honor my daughter Abigael. I want to thank my husband Robert for always being supportive and loving me even in my crazy. Thank you to my older son Daniel for always helping me laugh when I was so stressed out. A special thank you to Carlyn for making me a mom, changing my life for the better, and always being there for me when I did not love myself.

Table of Contents

Introduction

"Nobody can teach me who I am. You can describe parts of me, but who I am—and what I need—is something I have to find out myself."[1]
~Chinua Achebe

What is shit creek? The concept of being *up shit creek*, (without a paddle), is something everyone can relate to. As humans, we all have different problems, and life tests us in different ways. My first test started when I was born to a Vietnam veteran with severe post-traumatic stress disorder (PTSD) who joined a motorcycle club when I was young. But that same upbringing made me a nurse. I always flew by the seat of my pants, never really planning for life, just going with the flow of it, yet, always being reactive. I wasn't the kid who had my career path planned out. In fact, when I graduated high school pregnant, I had no idea the life I would go on to lead.

I feel very blessed, privileged, and honored to be a nurse, caring for so many people over the years. As a nurse, you see people when they are hurting and scared and full of questions about life and even death. We, as nurses, are the bridge between the patient, their diagnosis, and the doctor, often delivering bad news.

How does it make you feel when you have to just stand there as the physician explains there is nothing left to do for a family's loved one? You likely knew this conversation needed to happen, but it still is hard. As the nurse, your heart aches for the families. The patient may still be lying in the bed, hanging on, hooked up to

---

[1] https://quotefancy.com/quote/1005528/Chinua-Achebe-Nobody-can-teach-me-who-I-am-You-can-describe-parts-of-me-but-who-I-am-and

all the tubes and the machines. Death is so strange: family members are crying, or maybe just sitting there talking to the patient as if he or she will survive. Now, you are the one left with the patient's family to deal with the next step. It's up to you. It's your responsibility to be there for the questions like, *How did this happen?* You can see the fear of the unknown on their faces as they wonder what comes next. This is where you, the nurse, have to step up.

It's the nurse who has to ask, "What funeral home do you plan to use?"

How do you deal with the grief of telling family members that their loved one has passed, and, on top of that, having to ask at that moment about their final wishes? If you haven't had to ask this question to a grieving family yet, just wait, you will.

This is one of those moments, when the family may never remember your name but they will forever remember how you made them feel. Be the compassionate, understanding, and loving nurse they deserve, no matter how you feel. This moment is not about you, yet. That is how nurses have to function. We push aside our own feelings, but where does this stop?

We have to be able to manage these difficult situations and then walk out of that room and into the next patient's room without saying anything about the kind of day we're having because it's against HIPPA laws. We have to hold it in, wipe our tears, and move on to the next task. We get accustomed to bottling up or drinking down our emotions. Not being able to talk about our day has created trauma for nurses, and it is just one type of trauma nurses experience. We need to be able to discuss what we did, what happened to us during our shift, what we could have done better, and what we felt the doctors did or did not do for our patient.

Nursing school teaches you a lot about the mechanics of being a nurse. It prepares you to take the test to become a registered nurse, but it doesn't prepare you for the emotional trauma you experience from just going to work. I wrote this book to help you, as a nurse, navigate some of that trauma because I have lived it. I shared how I survived being a nurse over the last twenty years and all of the trauma I experienced in my life so you will know you can too.

It's against my internal code of ethics to hold all this in. It has started to feel as if hospitals and the government want emotionless nurses because of all the regulations and restrictions they put on us, but the very definition of *nurse* means to care for those who can't care for themselves, and that process involves emotions. These feelings need to be dealt with before they emerge as a drinking problem or something worse.

My reason for being a nurse has grown and transformed over the course of my career, but my deep desire to improve the world of nursing has never wavered. When I first learned about the founder of the nursing profession in nursing school, I wanted to be the next Florence Nightingale. I wanted to improve the nursing world, impacting it for good. I felt this fire start burning in me that I never quite understood until now. I want to make being a nurse the most sought-after profession. I want people to regard nursing with the sanctity it deserves, but that means we have to respect *ourselves* enough to seek healing, and then caring for our patients from a loving space not from a place of hurt or anger. There used to be such a high level of respect at the mention of being a nurse. It is such a beautiful career. We are there for patients when sometimes even their family cannot handle what has happened to them. They are not usually nice or in a good mood, but can you really blame them? We have the privilege to see people at their worst and give them hope.

Does this experience make most of us a bunch of cynical bitches? Yes. But we don't have to be. I can say that I was, for many years, a cynical, jaded, bitchy nurse. I now am calm and relaxed and do not let much get to me because I have learned techniques to release the trauma instead of keeping it in. I am going to describe these techniques throughout the chapters of this book. *Nobody* should be keeping that shit festering inside.

I used to be the nurse who would meet anyone for a drink after a crazy shift. But then, all the shifts were crazy, and we were drinking way too much. So, I had to find a different way to cope with the emotional trauma of being a nurse. I came to nursing with enough emotional baggage that I had no idea how to unpack or sort through, and I never expected my job to cause new trauma. We go into nursing for many different reasons, and the more I analyze my reasons, the core, deep-rooted reason that surfaces is that I truly enjoy helping others. At first, I thought I just wanted to save lives, but now I focus on helping others, including helping nurses learn to live happier lives and love being a nurse. There are five million nurses in the United States, and they need someone who understands what they are going through.[2] I want to nurse the nurses.

I hope to see all nurses love their jobs and help people get better, but for that to happen, nurses have to be brave enough to look at their own dysfunctional shit. While nurses are some of the strongest individuals I know, we also tend to avoid our own inner demons. Thankfully, instead of avoiding it, I reached a point when I realized I hated my life and needed a change. I thought if I changed *where* I was a nurse, then maybe things would be different, so I went from the ICU to the ER. That actually made me *more* cynical because I was seeing the raw and unfiltered side of society. Let me just put this out there: you ER nurses, *yes, you*, are a special brand of badass. You face things with a confidence that is unmatched in the nursing world. As a former ER nurse who had to have my boobs photographed by the police at work because I was kicked in the chest by a psych patient, I can say I know a thing or two because I have seen a thing or two.

As nurses, we all have our stories. I have people's faces ingrained in my memories, some for good reasons and some for

---

[2] https://www.consumershield.com/articles/how-many-nurses

bad. One night in the ER in a rough part of town that has a high poverty level, I cared for a little old lady who was not in her right mind. I walked her over to the toilet and had the EMTs who brought her in hold up sheets because she wouldn't let me close the door. She asked, "What's this hole for?" as she pointed to her groin.

And in my sassy nurse voice I said, "That's your vagina."

She said, "Oh, what's that for?"

I am sure every nurse has at some point had to explain to a patient what his or her body parts are for because as we age the mind doesn't work quite like it should.

Most of my experience in the ER was with treating adults, and that was hard enough. So, I want to take a moment to shout out to all the nurses who work with babies, neonates, and children. I commend you for the work you do. I knew myself well enough as a nurse to know I would not handle death in a child as well as an adult, so I stayed in mostly adult nursing. I have my own kids and do not handle them being sick that well, let alone having some kind of devastating disease. So, thank you for all you do.

That's the great thing about being a nurse, if you don't like where you are working, you can change it. It's not like working in any other profession: the possibilities are endless, but the pay sucks. I think we should get a standard hazard pay on top of our normal base rate. I mean, how many people go to work, get groped by their patients and don't think anything of it. Just the other day an older gentleman was tied down because he was swinging at the four of us trying to secure his NG tube with a bridle. I should have paid attention to where I was standing, but I just wanted to secure the tube before he dislodged it. So, I calmly said, "Sir, can you please stop grabbing my vagina." And, I cannot tell you the number of times I have gotten poop on me or been pooped on by patients over the years.

I can recall a specific patient that had C-diff, so thank goodness I had the gown on, but it only goes down so far. So, I rolled the patient away from me, and the other nurse was holding him on his side as I started to wipe. To my surprise, the patient let loose and exploded C-diff poop all over me, which ran down the yellow gown and my leg. I started to scream. I dropped my pants and yelled for someone to get me a new pair. Now, looking back, it was so funny. My coworkers were laughing at me in the moment. It has taken me a few years to find the humor, but now I can laugh at it.

As nurses, we see some really sad aspects of humanness. Being exposed to so much sadness takes a toll on you. So, I ask, *What are you doing to help protect your own sanity?* The answer is not to hide from it; it's not to shove it in a box and pretend you can just keep going. I will show you how to nurse yourself so you can do your job well and live well. Learning to fill your own cup before you start working as a nurse or early on in your career will help you to ward off feelings of burnout. Nurses give so much to their patients that they often feel empty by the end of the day. Giving from a full emotional cup allows you to not feel so depleted by the end of the 12 hours.

As a baby nurse, I did not have anyone to mentor me and guide me in self-care. I wish I would have; maybe it wouldn't have taken me so long to heal. But, then again, I wouldn't be who I am without all the trauma. And honestly, the healing process has made me a better nurse. I am more patient than I used to be. I can deal with dementia patients with more grace and without getting frustrated. I have learned to love on patients' families more than I used to because I understand nursing goes beyond the patient lying in the bed. Our care encompasses the patient's whole life situation. For instance, if your patient is constantly asking to leave but is nowhere near medically stable enough to be discharged, you inquire why he or she wants to leave. Most of the time, it's because the patient is a caregiver for someone else or has pets and no one to care for them. Being a nurse is a little like being a detective because you are helping the doctor figure out why the patient is here. Or you are actually the one to figure it out, but the doctor gets all the credit.

I have learned to see love in the everyday, even though I have suffered so much loss in such a short life. It did not happen overnight, but I promise you too can see the beauty in the gift you are to this world by being a nurse. I am here to show others that life is a fantastic experience and feeling the depths of grief can show you the boundless joy that life has to offer.

As you read my story, I hope you find the humor and the love and can see yourself healing along with me.

Chapter 1
Where it All Began

"Our lives are fashioned by our choices. First we make our choices. Then our choices make us."[3]
~ Anne Frank

My story starts at age 18. I was a rebellious smart-mouthed daughter. I was an only child who got everything she wanted. I was a brat. I had a miscarriage when I was 15 years old and was told I would never be able to carry a baby because of the scar tissue in my uterus. Because of this, I never took precautions against pregnancy. My senior year in high school, I was dating a 24-year-old guy who my mother set me up with. (It's OK if your eyes widen at this!) I could not ever think of setting up my 18-year-old daughter with a 24-year-old man. But she did, and we were great. Well, I didn't realize we were *not* until he told me I gave him a sexually transmitted disease (STD). I lost my shit. I was screaming at him that it wasn't from me. So, I went to my OBGYN and got tested. I was not infected with the disease he claims I gave him, but my doctor asked me if I was pregnant. I said "no."

He said, "We should test you just in case."

I peed in the cup and didn't think anything of it. Sure as shit, I was pregnant. Then, they did blood work to make sure the pee test was not a false positive, and I was definitely pregnant. So here I am, barely starting my life and already responsible for someone else. I was so happy because I never thought I would get to be a mom. My daughter turned out to be a prom baby. (My mother made

---

[3] https://quotefancy.com/quote/766593/Anne-Frank-Our-lives-are-fashioned-by-our-choices-First-we-make-our-choices-Then-our

sure to tell her that all the time.) I never saw being pregnant as a big deal, which is so crazy to me. I had so much childhood trauma from my parents that I wanted to feel loved by this baby so much. This child was my life, and I embraced being a mom. The sad part was I had not officially graduated high school yet.

The biological dad and I did not last long. I mean, I did not see the red flags early on but should have. For goodness' sake, he was cheating on me, which is how he got the STD (and I did not). And he already had a four-year-old daughter that he never saw and did not pay child support for, which should have been a red flag that he wasn't going to get the father of the year award any time soon. But what did I know? I thought I was in love.

He ended up getting fired from one job and bouncing to another. He was not in a good place, but he gave me my precious daughter, so I did not mind. He did end up asking me to marry him when I was around two months pregnant … but that was after he had held me hostage the day I told him I was pregnant. He refused to let me leave his house for hours, screaming at me that I had to get an abortion because he did not want to be a father again. The only way he let me leave was because I promised to get it done. I cannot explain the mental torture he put me through. Needless to say, I did not get it. The relationship only lasted a few months, and he quit talking to me around seven months pregnant. He did show up at the hospital to see her come into this world.

As for my dad, he was a very opinionated man. He did not speak to me until I was about four months pregnant. My mom had to tell him because of his PTSD and his explosive anger. He was so pissed at me. He said he had one job and that was to keep me from getting pregnant before graduation, and he failed. Well, yeah. *Hey Dad, if you hadn't been such an abusive, absent father, maybe I wouldn't have had so many daddy issues that caused me to use sex to feel loved?* (But, that's a whole different chapter.) He did not realize he was being abusive. He was just repeating the same type of parenting he was raised with because he never saw an issue with it. I hated it. I felt like I could never do anything right. I was always told children should be seen and not heard. And it was either his way or the highway. He would threaten to beat me then call the cops on himself and tell me how horrible a life I would have if that happened. It was like psychological warfare. But I can't even blame him totally because the shit he saw in Vietnam was horrific. I couldn't expect him to be loving and caring but that's what I needed. He did start therapy when I was a teenager and had gotten better, but dementia has taken that higher perspective away. Years later, he did better when he could. Funny that he was so pissed I had gotten pregnant, because when he saw that little girl, he was totally in love with her and being a grandfather.

I had such low self-esteem by the time I got pregnant. I know having Carlyn saved my life. That little girl did not know it, but her love saved my soul from utter destruction. She made me a mom. She is truly a God-given miracle that I never fully understood. I was so young when she was born that I did not understand the true miracle of getting pregnant and delivering a healthy baby. Now I do. Now I understand how many things have to line up perfectly so that the sperm can meet a healthy egg and produce a healthy child. I can only pray that someday I get to show her how much of a miracle she is to me. I will forever be grateful to God for making me a young mom. It was one of the hardest roads I have walked in my life, but it has been the most transformational. And I am a better person from being Carlyn's mom. Sadly, our mother-daughter relationship has been destroyed over the years, and she doesn't yet know how much I believe her existence saved my soul.

Today, I have a beautiful daughter who asked for some space until she feels ready to have a relationship with me, but after what we went through, I don't blame her. Unfortunately, she witnessed (and endured) so much trauma as a child—the same shit I went through but at a much younger age—giving her a whole different perspective as a child. I will get into that in a later chapter. It's a really long story.

Being a teen mom has so many universal challenges, especially being stared at and judged by older women. I read over 20 different baby books and made it my mission to be the best mom I could be. I learned how to breastfeed and was determined to stick with it, even though my mom did not breastfeed me and was not supportive at all. She kept trying to talk me out of it because it was hard. I refused. I wanted to give this baby everything she needed to be a happy and healthy girl, even though we were told she was going to be a boy from five different sonograms! (The quality was not as good back then.) My baby shower was for a boy, so Carlyn wore blue clothes for the first few months.

Trying to navigate life while still living at home with your parents *and* trying to be a mom—UGH!! It was so hard. My mom would not do what I wanted for my baby; she did what she wanted. It was mentally rough. My mom thought that since she raised me, she knew what she was doing. I thought, *Well, you fucked me all up, so sit down and be quiet. Give me a chance to make better decisions and not repeat your mistakes. OK? Thanks.* (I said I was a mouthy teenager.) I wasn't about to take advice from someone who, at that point, I felt had screwed me up beyond repair. I believe being a mom gave me the chance to give better than what I got as a child.

I had no idea how I was going to provide for this child. I did not have a job at the time. I was able to get assistance from the government and took John to court for child support. He did at least pay for that. Then, when Carlyn was four months old, we got a phone call that my dad was in a motorcycle accident and was being flown to Presbyterian Hospital in downtown Pittsburgh, the closest trauma center. We packed a few things and headed downtown.

We were not sure what we were going to see when we got to the hospital. My dad's life was hanging in the balance between life and death. He still had explosive anger issues from the war, and he always picked the bike club over being at my dance recitals. But I was still daddy's little girl. It was a weird dynamic because I never felt valued but always felt loved. I was still his only child, and we did everything together. Just the two of us would go to Kennywood, our local amusement park, and I helped him work on his motorcycle. Seeing him this way was gut wrenching for me. He was flown by a STAT MedEvac helicopter, and now, every time I see one in the air, I pray for the pilot, the crew, the patient, and the family. His crew was amazing. He was hit by a teenager making a left turn and flew over 20 feet, landing in some bushes. People saw it and called 911, which saved his life. He broke all but one of his ribs, shattered his right scapula, broke his left collar bone, and destroyed his left hand and wrist. They needed a cadaver bone to rebuild it.

Thank God, and I mean it! Thank the good Lord that he saved my father's head. No brain trauma. But, we found out that both lungs were punctured on the scene, and if that stat flight crew had not placed the chest tubes, he would have died. That's why I pray for them … because they saved my dad. My mom and I, along with Carlyn, spent the next week living in the hospital. They had a wing reserved for families from out of town, and it was a godsend. They even got Carlyn a crib so we could stay there. This is when I developed my love of intensive-care nursing. I admired those nurses for what they did for my dad and how well they cared for him. I knew what I was going to do with my life. I knew I wanted to help others the way these nurses helped us. I had some hurdles to overcome to be a nurse, but I knew that's what I wanted. My first hurdle was barely graduating high school. I had to take some classes to get my grades up before applying to nursing school, so I started with a biology class. I first applied to be a sonographer because I had done so poorly in high school from lack of trying that I did not think I would even get into nursing school. After the biology class, I saw that I was smart and went for nursing. I worked hard to get the grades that would get me into nursing school, and I learned so much. I had no idea of the incredible journey ahead.

I never would have guessed where my career would take me, but I am definitely thankful for the journey. I have always felt that everything happens for a reason. Things can happen *to* us or happen *for* us, but it is in our reaction that life happens. I used to be very reactive to life, but learning more about myself over the years, I have gained a sense of peace that life is happening *for* us. I have become more spiritual. I learned to meditate and quiet my mind. I believe in energy movement. I learned to see all sides of a situation before reacting. I have had to experience some terrible things to gain this knowledge, and I pray that reading this book helps you to gain some of these insights without having to experience the pain and suffering I did. This book is a great example of how you can learn from someone else's mistakes. It is also a great reflection of God's love for us. I believe I was being molded over the years into the human I am today, and without all that I suffered, I would not have become who I am. I can honestly say I am grateful for the lessons. I might have chosen a different way to learn them, but I am rather stubborn and opinionated. Just ask my ex-husband. I am sure he will agree.

Chapter 2
My Wedding to Dan

"A problem is only a problem when viewed as a problem. All change is hard at first, messy in the middle, and gorgeous at the end."[4]
~ Robin S. Sharma

I would like to place a disclaimer before you read this chapter: my ex-husband and I have a pretty decent friendship now. I think it's because we have been divorced longer than the number of years we were married. But, also, because we no longer hate each other. I would like to say how awesome he is now, and he has even acknowledged how he was a "real asshole" when we were married. We have both grown and changed so much. Now, you can enjoy the comical story of our wedding.

I got married young. The wedding had so many red flags; we should have never gone through with it. But then I wouldn't have two of my children, and I will never regret them. People who experience trauma usually feel it was their fault, taking on all the guilt. I did for years. I don't know if we traumatized each other or if we just each had so much childhood trauma from being raised by people who had a lot of their own unhealed wounds that we didn't know how to love each other. Or am I just trying to rationalize my past? I would swear my ex-husband was either a narcissist or just plain emotionally abusive, but I am not a doctor or a cop and have no right to formally call him those names. Now, I can see we were two young kids who each had our own childhood trauma that we

---

[4] https://quotefancy.com/quote/953678/Robin-S-Sharma-A-problem-is-only-a-problem-when-viewed-as-a-problem-All-change-is-hard-at

needed to heal. I will be honest: I *know* I was difficult to be married to because I had not healed any of my childhood trauma. I was still in survival mode mentally. Dan, my ex-husband, kind of helped raise me from being a spoiled little brat to being a wife and mom. I had no idea how to be an adult.

I know I will always love him for all the good things we survived together. He taught me so much, and I care about him as a human. I want him to be happy and have love in his life. I just have zero desire to ever see him naked again. *Not my job.*

When you do not take the time to heal your own inner child wounds, you end up hurting those around you. Have you ever heard the saying, *Don't bleed on those who did not cut you*? It is a very good visual reference to this theory. I think Dan and I were just too young and too wounded to ever work out. We each had our own issues and if we had actually done the work to heal them, maybe things would have been different. That's the question I always grapple with, *Would I change the things I went through because they are what made me be me?* My answer: I know I love who I am today.

I was only 19 when we decided to start dating. My ex-husband was the older brother of my high school best friend. We had hung out a ton and knew each other for years. In fact, he would have been at my daughter Carlyn's birth, but his sister did not wake him up when she was leaving to come to the hospital to see me. I remember I got a speeding ticket taking him to work when I was eight months pregnant, and the cop yelled at me that I was going to be a mom so I should have known better. I was 18. How was I supposed to know better? I was a baby having a baby.

I use the phrase "decided to start dating" because we were already friends. We knew a ton about each other. My dad had just gotten home a couple days before from the rehab place after his first motorcycle accident, and my mom said she would watch Carlyn so I could relax for a few hours. We both had done nothing but wake up and go see my dad for months. Dan was living with his sister at the time, and I was just going over to hang out with my best friend. I had *no intention* of leaving that night dating my best friend's brother. It was so taboo, especially since his mom hated me as his sister's friend.

I was the *bad influence* friend. I drove, and we would go to college parties. I took her to get her first tattoo. We each got a heart tattoo on the same spot on our legs, but mine has a bow, hers has a rose. She just never liked me being her daughter's friend. She sure wasn't going to like Dan dating me. He never listened to his mother's advice, so he did anyway. We really did not stand a chance of having a good marriage, did we?

I am an only child, and my mother spoiled me so much. I pretty much got anything I wanted, so I had an unlimited budget in my mind when planning the wedding. When I talked to Dan about picking a date to get married, he wanted an anniversary he could remember. He was a volunteer fireman, so 9-11 was an appropriate date to get married—just dial 9-1-1 for emergencies! He still has a pretty twisted sense of humor; seriously, just ask him. He is an ER nurse now and has seen some shit, and if you are also an ER nurse, you know what I mean. As an ER nurse, you use dark humor to deal with the crazy shit you see at work. I am a recovered ER nurse. I worked in it for a year and moonlighted for a few shifts here and there.

So the date was set, September 11, 1999. It was a beautiful fall day: not a cloud in the sky, warm but not so hot that the church was stuffy. I had made Dan promise not to be drunk for the ceremony. What do you think he was? Drunk before the wedding from doing shots with his brother and best man in the parking lot.

Like, are you for real?

I asked him to at least be sober when he said, *I do*. Nope, he couldn't do that. We had decided a few months before that we wanted to be newly pregnant for the wedding, so Carlyn would have a sibling. Well, turns out, I was six months pregnant because it only took one try. First try. And bam. Pregnant! They had to let out my wedding dress twice because I had gained so much weight. Come to find out, I birth really big babies. All four of them were huge.

After all the planning and prepping, the day was finally here. I was the biggest bridezilla ever. I made my bridesmaids wear matching hair clips, makeup, and shoes. I paid for them to have their hair done at the same place because I didn't trust them to match if they went elsewhere. I actually kicked out one of my bridesmaids for having an opinion. I decorated the hall myself that morning because I didn't trust anyone else. I did all the favors because I didn't trust the napkins to be tipped the right way. Bridezilla.

Back then, I did not have a name for the personality that comes out when I get stressed, but today I call her "crazy-packy lady." When I'm packing the car, this personality comes out in full force. But looking back, I can see that my over-controlling need to be in charge of everything comes from being let down too many times. I have trouble trusting others to live up to what they say because I had been let down by others so many times before. Yes, this is a trauma response. Crazy-packy lady still visits me, but I recognize her and can talk her down from the ledge.

Back then I had no control over her, and I was a wreck when I got stressed. There I was preparing for my wedding, six months pregnant, and I was a disaster. I had pretty much pissed off all my bridesmaids by the time the ceremony started. The preacher had warned me that there were to be no photos or video of the actual ceremony the day of the wedding. I was pissed. I told both my videographer and the photographer to "do whatever" I said because we were not coming back anyway, and the preacher was just a fill-in until the church got a new guy. I was already upset with him because we had to complete marriage classes, and the preacher told us we had no right getting married. HA HA HA. Funny how he ended up being right, but that's beside the point. I was determined to prove him wrong—maybe that's why we stayed married for way too long.

So, there we are standing before God and all our friends and family ready to pledge our love to each other, and the preacher says, "and the power of the Lord be with you."

And the lights go out.

Like are you for real? Was this real life? What just happened?

This was the first direct sign from God that maybe we should not be doing this. (We now laugh at this point in the video, knowing that we got a divorce, but seriously.) As we continued the ceremony, he said something else about *the power of the Lord*, and the power came back on. I wish I would have understood what it means to follow my intuition back then, but I wouldn't have my amazing daughter Abby if I had, so it's OK. She is my prize for being married to Dan. I was already pregnant with our son, Dan, who is the golden child. He was the first boy to be able to carry on the last name, and Abby was born a few years later.

The flickering lights were not even the biggest red flag. After the ceremony, we went to a park for pictures. I had insisted that everyone in the wedding party go by limo, but our party was so huge that we had two limos. Dan and I, his brother and his girlfriend, and his sister and her soon-to-be husband were in the first limo. The best man, maid of honor, and the other two bridesmaids and groomsmen were in the second limo. By the time we got to the park 20 minutes away, the second limo was completely out of liquor. During pictures, they actually got into our limo and snatched some of ours. We didn't know that then.

While we were at the park, my little cousin from my mom's side, an ornery junior groomsman, was throwing acorns and hitting someone, so Dan picked him up, sat him on a bench and told him to knock it off. We went about getting our pictures and headed to the reception.

When we arrived at the reception, we were greeted by one of Dan's EMS friends who was looking for the best man because his wife was in the bathroom in active labor. Thank goodness all of his family was also invited to the wedding because he was so drunk that he couldn't drive her to the hospital. His best man jacket was given to a guy who looked like a linebacker from the Steelers so he could give the best man speech instead. The best man was an average size. It does make for a funny part in the video as everyone was singing the song from the movie *Tommy Boy*, "fat guy in a little coat."

At the reception, my little cousin told his dad, my uncle, that Dan had "beat him" when we were getting pictures. Instead of talking to us to see what really happened, my uncle and like ten members of my mom's side of the family got up and just left. It took a while to realize with all the other chaos going on.

Remember when I said the group in the other limo drank all the liquor and was completely smashed? Well, the groomsman from the second limo, who was my best friend, called Dan's mom a bitch, so Dan punched him and was about to beat on him, until a bunch of people pulled him off. I had no idea a fight had even broken out. Someone called the cops. I was six months pregnant, and I was so upset talking to the cops. Dan almost went to jail. The rest of my mom's side of the family left because the groomsman Dan fought was dating my cousin.

The most devastating part of the day for me was when I was standing outside with the cops and the drunken groom, when my then father-in-law came over and, putting his arm, around me said, "Well, you're a true Furlong now. You got the cops invited to your party!"

The red flags were all over the place. I did not pay attention to a single one. I honestly did not even realize back then that I was not in a healthy relationship. I had never been taught boundaries. I did not know what self-respect was, nor did I have any.

When you are in an unhealthy relationship because you never learned how to love yourself, it's easy to stay. Once you realize that you are worth so much more and deserve to be loved, the way you need to thrive, that's when life gets good. You have to make the decision to put your own self first. It is not an easy transition. The process of changing your mindset and breaking all the old thinking habits is difficult, but it is so worth it.

I started loving myself a little bit at a time over a 12-year journey. It is about being consistently better than the version of yourself from the day before. No one can make huge changes all alone and have them stick. I have had a few life coaches over the years. Changing your entire mindset from lack, low self-esteem, and feeling useless and worthless to knowing you are a child of God created to *be* loved and to *give* love takes dedication. Do not ever let anyone make you feel bad for improving your life. I lost a lot of so-called friends in this process, but if they were true friends, they would have supported me.

The wedding was a disaster, but the whole marriage was not so bad. We grew up together. Dan pushed me through school. I would never have gotten four semesters of straight As, made it on the dean's list, and received a full scholarship to finish my bachelor's degree if he had not told me I wasn't smart enough or how I wasn't able to do something. I used that negative attention to push me to be better. But my unstable hormonal self must have been horrible to be married to. He never knew who he was coming home to. Was I going to have dinner ready or scream at him when he walked in the door? Remember, we were married before cell phones were a normal thing.

I did try marriage counseling, but Dan hated the therapist, so it did not work. My biggest takeaway from the time I was married to him was that it taught me what not to do to be a good wife. So, all the things I used to do I no longer do. I like to think of it as my training ground, which helped me become a better wife for the soul mate I was going to meet.

I know we are in rough waters right now, but stick with me. There are calmer waters ahead.

With all due seriousness, if you are in an abusive relationship—and yes, verbal abuse counts—do not stay. There is help. I have provided a list of resources in the back of the book to help you. I am happy I went through all that I did because I used all of the hurt as stepping stones into the life of blessings I have now. I truly see each obstacle as an opportunity to improve. This was one of the first mindset shifts I started to make, and it is a very useful tool for healing.

Chapter 3
The Blended Family

"Do the best you can until you know better. Then when you know better, do better."[5]
~ Maya Angelou

The years between the divorce (2011) and losing my mom (October of 2013) are still pretty painful to think about because it forces me to face the poor decisions I made—ones I feel destroyed my relationship with my oldest daughter, Carlyn. I was a selfish person back then. I did not know or understand self-care. All I knew was that I was not happy. I ended up leaving Dan for a *manchild*. He was a little younger than me, but mentally he was still a child. I did not realize because he lied to me so much. He told me so many stories I truly do not know what was the truth. I just knew that at that moment in my life, God used him to get me on the right path.

While I was married to Dan, I was drinking a lot, and sometimes I would even drink until *blackout drunk* level. I was not being a good mother at all. I truly believe God used Antonio to help fix me because he told me, "If you want to date me, you have to quit drinking." My drinking was so bad that I got drunk at EMS weekend—a celebration of EMS personnel and an education conference held yearly at Seven Springs (a local ski resort)—and gave a guy a blow job who wasn't my current husband. I was acting like a whore without any cares in the world instead of a mother who should have protected her children. I don't really remember all the details. They are really fuzzy. That was pretty much the end of that

---

[5] https://www.somethinkofvalue.com/maya-angelou-quotes/

marriage. I was in such a self-destructive mode, but I did not care. I don't think I even cared about being alive.

I was in such a space of self-loathing. I definitely did not have any self-respect. Everything was a wreck. My marriage was over. My finances were shitty. Dan and I filed for bankruptcy, but getting divorce negated the bankruptcy filing. The bankruptcy court discharged us, making it null and void. I was working three jobs to try and save the house so the kids did not have to move schools, but the fighting and the hatred were so much. I know I hurt Dan, and for that, I am truly sorry. And have told him that. I still have lots of regrets I am working through, but then, I play the mental game of, *If I regret how I became me, then do I regret me?* I do not regret who I became out of all of this.

After the divorce, (and in the middle of my mess) I decided to let my new boyfriend move in with me. I did not realize how stupid it was to try to blend a family when there was so much strife. It was a poor decision.

Blending a family is hard in any situation. It is twice as difficult when there are estrangement issues for various reasons. When you fall in love, you think your love can handle anything, but honestly, love and maintaining a relationship are different beasts. Reality is not as pretty as the movies make you believe it is. Maybe that's why our society loves to read romance novels. We all want to believe that someday our Prince Charming is going to sweep us off to a castle and our lives will be magical. They give us this false sense of what love is supposed to be—this lustful desire to want to rip each other's clothes off all the time.

Real love, the daily stuff that us normal people (not movie stars) need to accept, is not that kind of romance. It is still passionate, just not that glamorous. It is the little things. It's when he grabs your hand while driving to the grocery store and kisses it. It's finding matching socks and making dinner for your husband as he gets ready for the extra shift he picked up so the kids can keep going to gymnastics. Love is family. Family is not always the mom, the dad, and their biological kid(s) anymore. It would still take me a few more years to find this kind of love.

This new blended family of yours-mine-and-ours (sharing children as stepparents) is the true testament of God's love. God made our hearts big enough to love beyond the traditional family structure, and I sure turn to him for love and strength while blending our family now, which science says it takes seven years to fully do.[6]

When I first tried to blend families—with the *manchild* I left Dan for—there was the dramatic teenage girl of 14, the 12-year-old son who assumed the man-of-the-house role, the 7-year-old princess, and me, the overworked momma. I came to this situation with an overbearing mother and father (who babysat a ton) and an ex-husband who had never been a great father to his children. The *ex* always felt children should be seen and not heard in his younger years.

Then there was the new boyfriend (slide in any name—the personality is usually the same—because until you do the inner work, ladies, you will keep attracting the same shitty men) and his child, who was four years old. And if it were as simple as us learning how to get along and respect each other, it would have been a cake walk, but in reality, well, it was uglier.

But that's not all! Then, there was my ex-husband's new girlfriend, who had three kids of her own and an ex-husband. So, you would have thought we could have been friends because we had similar stories, but, for whatever reason, she did not want that. She was full of opinions of how the divorce should work and how the custody should be. With so many extra children now in the mix, my kids had to compete for attention at both homes. I did not realize it was an issue until years later. If I would have understood how this hurt my kids, I would have made different decisions. I regret not sending them to individual therapy. That is the major recommendation I give all parents going through divorce is to put your child(ren) in child-appropriate therapy to help process all the

---

[6] https://www.gottman.com/blog/stepping-back-to-save-my-stepfamily/

emotions that come up in divorce, and so they know it was not their fault and they are so loved by both their parents. Sadly, adults do not always do what's best for their child(ren). I was not making good decisions to help my children grow into amazing adults. They managed to do that despite what they went through.

Then, of course, there was my ex-husband's extended family—his brother and his wife, who never liked me in high school. Honestly, I never liked her either. My ex-husband's sister is also my ex-best friend, which complicated the situation. The ex-in-laws would bash and badmouth me every holiday and make my youngest cry; she was there to see her dad, not to hear about how everyone hates her mother. Why do adults think children need to hear their opinions about the ex-spouse? I just do not understand. Opinions are like assholes; every human comes with one. And they made sure to voice all their opinions while we were trying to blend families.

I made sure to *not* talk shit about my ex to the younger ones because no matter how I felt about him, he was still their father and deserved to have a relationship with them. Back then, I did not think Carlyn would ever want a relationship because she had always said how much she hated him, but I think that might have been a child trying to validate her mother's feelings because now she loves him and doesn't speak to me. But who knows what she was thinking because I never made her go to therapy like I did. I tried, but she refused. I should not have given her a choice. Also, I knew they would develop their own opinions of him as they got older, and they have as adults. And thank the good Lord they all have some kind of relationship with him.

Now I have to be honest. I was living with my new boyfriend way too early—in my defense, I did not know any better back then. And he was the guy I admitted to cheating on my husband with and who I left my husband for. So, understandably, their opinions of me, what I did, and how I went about it were most likely valid. But they absolutely did not and should not have been voiced to my children.

They deserved to spend time with their extended family without hearing smack about their mom.

But wait, there's more. Then throw in the mix the new boyfriend's overbearing, overprotective mother, plus, his ex-girlfriend (who we referred to as Baby Mama Drama) had her own overbearing mother. She also voiced her opinion about how we should be raising our kids. We cannot forget that Baby Mama Drama also had a live-in boyfriend.

So, blending a family is way more complicated than it initially looks. It takes so much work and communication for a blended family to truly develop the sense of being a family. Having all these other people in your relationship makes it difficult, especially when no one understands healthy boundaries and each person I mentioned comes with their own unhealed childhood trauma. This relationship was doomed from day one. Thank you, Lord, for the lessons, but I am also so thankful for unanswered prayers. Have you ever begged God for something and was told No, only to then realize it was the best thing for you? That was this relationship for me. I have tons of letters I wrote to God begging him to make things work and let me be happy. I am so blessed to have had so many unanswered prayers or Nos from God.

I am grateful for all that I learned from it, though. I learned that I have the rare ability to see things from all angles. I came to see how the choices Baby Mama Drama made about visitation and child support affected my boyfriend and how we blended our kids. I saw how hard it was from the father's perspective, and thus, how my decisions affected my ex-husband and his ability to blend our kids with his new girlfriend's kids.

Different parenting styles, including ideas on how or when to punish kids, bring up the challenges of blending individual morals.

Who babysits while you're working? Do I let my new significant other babysit? Do I treat them like another parent?

Do I let them discipline my children? Do I set ground rules? How does this all work? Some families do this effortlessly. Some, like ours, struggled.

I said from the beginning that everything happens for a reason. God puts us where we need to be to grow and learn the skills for his next adventure for us.

I can say that I am on an incredible journey home to God, and I love how he shows me he is working in my life. God used this failure to blend these families and prepare me for the best in life. God has never let me down, even when I felt I was failing at life. I could see his hands working in me as I started to learn to love myself.

Since I was a little girl, I always felt a desire to help others. It is the gift that God gave me. I want to make big changes for the better in the world before I leave it. Not like world peace or feeding the hungry, but through this book. Maybe some mom reading this will come to know and understand herself a little better. I write this in hopes that one person opens her eyes to what God is showing her every day as he is right there loving her.

My most favorite story of how God makes every decision of ours count is about a normal day for the ex-boyfriend and me. We both worked steady night turn. I am a nurse with her PHRN, and my ex was an EMT, so we would get the kids off to school and then sleep and cuddle. That was our time. For Christmas, his mother bought him a remote starter for his truck. On this particular day, we drove out to the shop that was installing it with both our vehicles so I could drive him home. I followed him to the shop to drop off his truck. I drove home, and we let the dogs out and went to sleep. A normal routine for us. A coworker asked us to listen on our radio that day, and if there was a bad call to please come help her. Her partner that day was not the brightest star in the sky. We worked on the ambulance together in the same town we lived in, so it was easy for us to do this.

My ex-boyfriend knew I hate boogers. I know, gross part, but focus with me. Around 1 p.m., we got the call that his truck was done. I drove to the shop, while he sat in the passenger seat pretending to pick his nose and wipe it on my shoulder, but I had no idea he was just pretending. I thought he was actually wiping boogers on my shoulder. I was so grossed out and pissed off that I pulled my truck over as I yelled at him. I got out and frantically wiped my shoulder, yelling and dancing around the truck for a few seconds, while he was laughing hysterically at me.

I was done and so frustrated with him, but as I got back in my truck, the radio went off for an unresponsive male who wasn't breathing about two blocks away from where we were. You better believe we got serious fast. I flipped the truck around and hauled ass to the address. We radioed our friend on the ambulance crew to let them know that we were a few minutes out and on the way. We arrived to a very brittle diabetic who was barely holding onto life. Then, we assisted in saving his life. When the call was all said and done, our friend thanked us so much for being there because she knew her partner could not handle bad calls.

My ex-boyfriend learned a valuable lesson that day. I had been trying to explain that everything happens for a reason: God allowed him to act gross so I would pull over and take those few extra minutes, putting me in the right place at the right time to save a life. That right there is how I make a difference in this world. To me, this man was a patient who had taken too much insulin and had not eaten enough, but, to his family—who watched us move swiftly to place an IV, give medications and oxygen, and check his blood sugar to make sure it came up—he was a husband, a father, a grandfather, and a loving member of their family.

So, even when you think what you do doesn't matter, it does because your course of action sets in motion another action that causes something else to occur, and so on. Like the concept that if you go back in time and change something, you would effectively change the whole trajectory of your life. Being aware of your greater purpose in this life helps make all the stress worth it. My ex-boyfriend said that being with me and helping me raise my kids in those years made him a better father. God knows what he is doing, and he works all things for our good. We need to believe that and let him do his wonderful work in our lives.

I know my time with that boyfriend taught me a lot about how to love, but the biggest lesson I learned from that relationship was when he left me the same way I left my ex-husband. It was a dish of karma that I knew I deserved. What I did not expect was a moment between my ex-husband and me that changed our relationship and how we functioned as a former couple trying to be good parents together but separate. He came to help me when we were getting kicked out of our home. In that moment, I apologized, and he forgave me for everything. We talked for hours at what used to be our kitchen table, and it was a pivotal moment, though it was still rocky, and we still disagreed on a lot.

Blending families is so much harder than being a biological parent. Having a child of your own is hard. I do not underestimate those struggles, but loving someone else's child is so much harder. You have to actively remind yourself that they are just a child who doesn't know any better than what they are taught. Children are, in my opinion, mostly a product of their environment. Think back to a time when you yelled at your child, or said *that phrase* and you thought to yourself, *Oh my goodness, I turned into my mother or my father.* Every parent has said it, and if you haven't yet, just wait. You will. I caught myself saying the, "You keep crying, I will give you something to cry about," comment. My father used to say this all the time. He also felt that children should be seen and not heard. You do what you're taught … until you realize there are better options. Then you can learn and do better.

Now, there are cases when children are in such a bad place that they work twice as hard to be the opposite of what they saw growing up. I saw that type of parenting from my parents. They both had siblings, so they did not want any for me. My mother and father had agreed that because they had strict rules growing up, they would do the opposite for me. I had no rules, no guidance, and no real supervision after the age of ten. They fed me and gave me anything I wanted, but for discipline, I was pretty much self-taught, which was not a great idea. I was known for my house parties as a teenager.

That, in my opinion, was the wrong choice. I go with the research-driven theory that children thrive on being held accountable for their actions and that kids like to please their parents. I had the luxury of taking many psychology classes while working for my bachelor's degree, including child psychology classes that my parents never had. I thought I was trying to use sound theory. I thought by being strict and making my kids accountable they would have a better childhood than I felt I did. Sadly, I feel it caused my oldest daughter to resent me. So, I stopped using the theory, and I realized we are all just flying by the seat of our pants—no one really has a clue. Neither of my parents went to college. My father spent many years just barely holding on to his job because of his anger issues, which were finally diagnosed as PTSD from the war. His drinking ruined my childhood. Please do not underestimate my love for my parents; I just do not happen to agree with how they chose to raise me.

When you're blending families, you have all the history from your own childhood mixed with everything from your significant other's childhood and all the families. Then, we're trying to navigate all we know from childhood and parenting experiences of our own, and we get the title of "stepparent." That really bothers me. A "step" is something we walk on. I know that many stepchildren *do* tend to walk all over their parents, so in those cases, the word fits. For my ex-boyfriend and me, we used "other mother" or "other father" because we were still helping to raise each other's children, and we did not ever want to replace the child's love for their biological parents. *But,* we did feel that we deserved better than being "stepped on." The ex-boyfriend's "other mother" is who taught him this theory.

His parents divorced when he was only two years old. All he ever knew was having "other" parents. I come from a very traditional mom, dad, and child home. All my friends growing up had parents who were married and lived as "one happy family." So I was flying by the seat of my pants and holding on tight to this "other mother" role.

I can remember the first time my seven-year-old referred to my ex-boyfriend as her "other father." We had agreed early on that when we moved in together, we would not force the children to call us anything but our first names. We wanted to respect the children, their choice, and their comfort level.

My ex-boyfriend's son, Andrew, was only four, so during the school year, we got to see him every day from 3 p.m. to 8 or 9 p.m. It was awesome. On this particular day, my ex-boyfriend was at home with my older two, and I took the younger two to the grocery store to get something to make for dinner. Everyone has seen those double-driver huge toy shopping buggies for the kids that are a nightmare to drive through the store. Most days I would say "No," but that day, I let them get in it. I lifted Andrew up and helped Abby climb in. She was just starting to enjoy being the big sister instead of the baby. She buckled his seat belt, then hers, and we were off. I was going down my grocery list as they were playing and pretending to drive the cart; meanwhile I held the cart in place with my foot on the wheels, while trying to reach for apples. They were talking, and Abby caught my attention with, "Momma, does Andrew have two mommies like I have two daddies?"

I froze for a second. I had no idea how to answer. Now, keep in mind that I was trying not to let the kids know that right at that moment, and I thought my heart had truly stopped.

My ex and I had discussed what we would want the kids to call us, but we did not realize how soon it would be. When you're in love with someone, you have all these wonderful grand plans, but then life happens. We got into the daily juggle of school, work, dinner, chores, homework, dance lessons, and Boy Scouts, and we seemed to have forgotten the most important part of being parents—we never talked to the kids.

Finally, I answered with, "Yes, I guess he does now, doesn't he?" And we moved on to the next aisle.

That question was the first time it occurred to me that my life was never going to be—*nor could it ever be*—the way it was when I was raised. And, I was scared. OK, I was horrified, but I made it through the store. That day, I realized I needed a new set of standards and some new theories on raising kids.

It wasn't until we split up that I started really changing and growing myself. One of the important lessons I learned from this experience is that it's OK to be dysfunctional when you don't know any better, but as soon as you know better, do better. For me, the first step toward knowing better and doing better was that I started going to therapy.

Antonio did something for me the day I almost took my own life, and I will always be grateful for that. Antonio and I had a fight. And I was fighting with Dan in court … and out of it. He was not being a good dad. I was struggling to make enough money to pay the mortgage, and he kept refusing to let me refinance the house without him—I was mentally exhausted. I had a lump in my throat, and the nurse in me feared the worst. I had gone in to work in downtown Pittsburgh. It was in February. There was ice on the river, and it was so cold out. I tried to get into the building, but it was locked. I could not find a way in. I had parked by PNC Park, the baseball stadium across the river from the office, and walked because I did not know how to read a bus schedule yet and all the parking close to the building was full. I was so mentally distraught from my life being a disaster that I broke. I mentally just broke when I couldn't get into the building to get to the work that needed done. I was already certain that my boss hated me. She talked about me to other coworkers very loudly near me so I could hear her. As all the negative thoughts piled on, I truly felt that my kids would be better off without me. I called Antonio crying—full-body sobbing, hysterically crying. I walked, crying like that, looking like a true mental patient, across the Clemente Bridge. I walked down by the river and stared at the water for a long time.

I thought to myself, *It's cold enough. I could just jump in and freeze to death.*

When I said that aloud on the phone, Antonio rushed to me and stopped me. I know that was God working. God still had plans for me.

Antonio pointed out that I was actually standing about 50 yards from the river patrol, and they would have saved me, so it was a shitty plan. But something changed in me that day. When I got home, my mom was there, watching my kids. I cried and hugged her. I thought I hit rock bottom that day. Turns out, I was far from rock bottom, but again, stay with me. There are calmer waters coming.

All of these lessons were shaping me to be the best version of myself, and I would need it for what lay ahead. The second lesson I learned through trying to blend our families is that parenting is not standard at all. Blending families takes great communication skills, and healthy boundaries are a must. Being able to hear difficult things and have tough conversations is critical. Learning to tell your kids you are sorry for the mistakes you made is a big one, and forgiveness is achievable. And always be willing to love.

Chapter 4
My Hell Year

"Life is short and unpredictable. Eat the dessert first!"[7]
~ Helen Keller

A series of events in my twenties tipped off my need to completely change who I was.

In 2009, I was working as an ICU nurse in the local hospital I had been at since I left the Veterans Affairs (VA). Now, 20 years later, it really stings that I left the VA because if I had stayed, I would be retiring with a full federal pension at 46 years old, but I also wouldn't be who I am. I was feeling pretty confident as an ICU nurse, and I was even in charge sometimes. I had earned my CCRN. I had received my BSN, and I was applying to go to FNP school. You needed to work as a nurse for five years before grad school would even look at you.

Back in my day (lol) we had to take grad school entrance exams, have community service experience, and complete a list of other things for them to even look at your application. Now, hell, they don't even wait till you pass the NCLEX to try and get you signed up for a MSN program. Personally, I feel you need the five years of experience to understand how a hospital works, but maybe I'm just *old school*. It takes 10,000 hours to be considered an expert and that adds up to a little over five years working the three 12-hour shifts. I mean, *why wouldn't you want a nurse practitioner who was only an RN for a couple months before entering the MSN 18-month program to be a CRNP to prescribe you life-saving medications!* There's no reason not to trust her opinion, right?

---

[7] https://quotefancy.com/quote/822699/Helen-Keller-Life-is-short-and-unpredictable-Eat-the-dessert-first

Personally, I would want a nurse practitioner that was a nurse for ten years before going to grad school … but that's just me.

When I was working as an ICU nurse, I was not doing well mentally. I was diagnosed with Hashimoto's disease by a resident in the ICU.

I was at work one day when Dr. Tishmal said, "Come here."

I replied, "Why?"

I swear he had a girlfriend on every floor. Most of the residents did back then. The one I flirted with the most was Dr. Hottie. Oh man, he was cute. I think I just loved the attention since I wasn't getting it at home.

But anyway, I went over to him, and he said, "Turn around," and he put his hands on my neck and said, "Swallow."

I did.

He said, "Have you ever had your thyroid checked." When I replied that I hadn't, he said, "Go get it checked."

Turns out I had an underactive thyroid. Anytime someone would ask about my thyroid, I would always joke, "It's probably cancer. They just didn't find it yet." Needless to say, I knew NOTHING of the Law of Attraction back then. If I did, I would not have spoken that into existence. Now, I guard my words carefully.

Hormonally, I was off balance. My soul was crying out for more, for something. She felt trapped. She felt like her life was being snuffed away like a candle. At home, I was miserable. I needed to feel something. I needed to feel passion, to feel anything, and I would beg Dan to love me. I would cry and tell him I needed more; I needed something from him to feel loved. I think it was my inner child crying out for understanding and to be with my soulmate. I was in this constant state of searching. Dan used to tell me I was nuts and crazy all the time. He would say I was bipolar. He had no medical degree to make these assumptions, but he was great at being condescending. He almost made it an art form; I hated my home life.

So, when a guy at work would flirt with me, I loved it. I craved that kind attention because in that moment, I had a tiny piece of feeling wanted, and I just wanted to feel wanted. But I still had three kids at home, and I knew divorce would hurt them. I had no idea just how much or in what ways. I did not want to destroy my marriage because I wanted to be a good mom. The self-loathing was intense. I had no idea of the generational trauma I was carrying internally.

I struggled with wanting a divorce for about four years. I was in an internal battle, believing that I deserved to be happy, but then I would remember that I signed up to be a mom. I knew I should put my kids first. I watched my mom give up her entire life so I could have a better one and thought that's what a good mother does. *A good mom suffers for the sake of her children.* I was so wrong, but it was a starting point. My inner queen was forcing her way to the surface.

I felt torn. I felt incomplete. I always felt as if a part of me were missing. I didn't know back in 2009 that I would transform my life, and I would find that missing piece.

I had gotten into such a rut in the ICU dealing with the same types of patients over and over. I did not feel like my brain was being challenged anymore. I was searching for the feel-good hormones that the adrenaline rush of caring for critically ill patients gave me. I was picking up extra shifts, working Monday through Friday daylight shifts in the ER and maintaining my weekend program in the ICU for the last year of my time at UPMC. I was constantly looking for the thing to make me feel satisfied. So, I started studying for my PHRN exam, which is the nationally certified paramedic exam. It would give me the ability to work on the ambulance. I was always chasing the adrenaline. I did not understand at the time that happiness came from within. I feel it was God preparing me to help others on their journey to discover their authentic selves.

I was enjoying my career, but I was still struggling as a mom. I still did not realize that I was not with my kids enough. I was so exhausted from all the stress, so even on my days off, I wasn't available emotionally. On my days off, I was home, and I would make dinner, but having a clean house was never really a priority for me. I knew my family deserved a clean home, though, so I did the least amount necessary. I tried, but I sucked as a housewife. The only time I did a deep clean was to host a candle party.

Then in July of 2010, my life hit a wall. Looking back, it was definitely my higher self trying to get my attention, but I was a seriously stubborn bitch. I was working on the ambulance full-time as a PHRN (aka paramedic) but started as a nurse, plus working as a nurse full time in the ER, plus going back to school for my master's. I was diagnosed with Crohn's disease back in 2003 while in nursing school. I was one of those students. (Chuckle.) I went to my PCP and said, "I have all the symptoms of colon cancer. I have the stringy poop, constipation, and severe abdominal pain." My doctor thought I was crazy but scheduled me for a colonoscopy. I got it done at Mercy Hospital because my mother-in-law at the time worked in the ICU at Mercy and loved the gastroenterologist there. I can vividly remember him telling me that he was very sorry, but I had Crohn's disease, and I was elated. I was so happy I did not have colon cancer in my 20s. After that, I never really had any problems … until I started to cheat on my husband while working two full-time jobs and smoking and drinking a lot. The stress was just too much. I had developed horrible belly pain to the point that Dan had to carry me into the ER (where I worked) to be seen.

I spent four days in the hospital as a patient because the Crohn's disease was so flared up from being under so much mental and emotional stress. Even as a nurse, I did not fully understand how much stress affected my organs. I never realized what this probably did to my kids. Their mom was not invincible. I went from being the nurse to being the patient. I did try to have fun with my sick, twisted sense of humor. I would push my IV pole down the hall and go visit my friends working in the ICU so much that they marked me a wandering risk.

Dan was a car salesman for the longest time, and we made good money. But he gave that all up to become an EMT and enrolled in nursing school. At the time of this flare up, he and I were actually working Sundays together. He was my EMT on the ambulance. In fact, if our dumb asses wouldn't have spent it all, we would be millionaires at this point in our lives. We were making six figures back in 2008–2010 but didn't save a penny. We lived. We bought the kids so much stuff. We had a pool and season passes to Sandcastle, our local swim park. We ate out a freaking ton. We also worked a lot. It was no wonder I got burned out. I always wonder if our working together helped destroy our marriage faster or if it was just all part of the plan.

From 2010–2012, I was under so much stress, fighting with Dan (we fought a lot) and arguing with my mom over how to raise my kids. She never respected me as a mother. My kids would tell me that when I walked out of the house to go to work my mom would say, "OK, she's gone. We can do xyz …"—whatever it was that I had just told them they were not allowed to do. It's no wonder my children never respected me. The two most influential people in their lives—their dad and their grandmother—did not show me any respect, so why did I expect them to? I did not think I could truly get across the depths of my despair during this time.

It was Christmas 2010 when Dan got incredibly drunk at his sister's house, and I had enough. We always had these kinds of screaming matches—full-on psycho matches. Again, I didn't realize it then, but we were so toxic as a couple. We were and are great as friends, but the marriage was just not good. Over the next two years, we fought over child support and who was going to get what in the divorce. He finally moved out, and for a few days, I wasn't sure if I had made the right decision. I was already dating someone else, which was a huge mistake, but there were lessons to be learned. I believe that God used Antonio to get my attention, as I mentioned in the last chapter, because I can remember the day we decided to start seeing each other before Dan and I split up.

I wanted a way out of my marriage so badly that I was willing to do anything, even stop drinking so I could have a boyfriend as an excuse to leave. I feel God used this moment to save me from the alcoholic I was becoming. I now had to learn new coping skills because I could not drown my sorrows in a bottle anymore. Thank God I was in therapy already.

By the time June came around in 2012, I was working three jobs trying to keep my house with a monthly mortgage payment of almost two thousand four hundred dollars. I was working as a paramedic at two different stations and as a full-time ICU nurse. I was never at home, always at work. Thank God my mom was able to raise my children at that time. I was struggling so much in every aspect of my life. I thought I had hit rock bottom. But still, I had not yet.

The hardest months of my life started in June 2012 when I was heading to an interview in Monroeville, a suburb east of Pittsburgh, for a nurse supervisor position. I really wanted that position, since I felt like it was my time to move up in the nursing world. I waited so long, and I was so happy. I was driving my Hummer H3, with a stick shift, so it took a few extra seconds to get going when the light turned green (which actually saved my life). I loved that truck. I was sitting at the intersection of Route 30 and Robbins Station Road. It was an intersection where Robbins Station is on a little hill, a slight elevation in relation to the four-lane highway I was turning onto. It is like you are looking down onto the major roadway from this little backroad. It was not a clear site to turn on to. I was the first car in line and sitting in neutral while putting my makeup on because I was never on time. My truck was my makeup room. My coffee was sitting next to me. (I was one of those coffee snobs who had to have the perfect flavored creamer and the right amount of sweetener.) I hadn't even gotten to take a sip yet. As the light turned green, I pressed in the clutch, put the truck in first gear, and started to pull out. I had just crossed onto Route 30, and BAM. I got hit. My life as I knew it was over in that instant.

I recall an intense pain and weird feeling in my head. I guess I blacked out from hitting my head, and I woke up to OnStar yelling at me, asking me how many people were in the car, and if I was OK, repeatedly, until I answered.

I could not figure out how I had gotten all the way across the road and was now facing the road I just drove down. I was so confused. All I could think of was my kids. Thank God my mom was watching them. Because I still worked at Irwin EMS, I found out from friends at the EMS station that my accident was called in as a rollover. So, when the 911 operator dispatched, they believed my truck was on its roof. My H3 was spinning on two wheels, which caused the sensor to detect a rollover, notifying OnStar. Some asshole in a super-duty work truck that was from a local car dealership blew the red light. There was a four-second delay for my light to turn green after his light turned red, and he still plowed right through me. The driver never even tried to stop. No skid marks at all.

I thank the Good Lord, because if it were not my guardian angels and the powers above, I would have been dead that day. God used those four seconds to save me. I think it's because I have a higher purpose than just going to work and paying my bills. I believe we all have a higher purpose than just surviving. I have something that I still need to give to this world, and it has not been fulfilled yet. I feel we each have a unique gift we are meant to give the world, and I am so grateful to be alive and for the opportunity to spread the good news.

This moment in my life helped define who I am today. I did not realize it for a few weeks, but that truck almost killing me sparked a change in me. It fanned the flame that was sparked those few months before when I asked Dan, "Is this really all there is to life?"

Immediately after the crash, I rode in an ambulance to a trauma center with the one medic at North Huntingdon EMS that I did not get along with when I worked there. They knew my truck, so they knew who they were coming to rescue that day. I was currently dating the guy I cheated on my ex-husband with (finally getting that divorce I wanted!) but when that truck hit me, and I was unconscious for a few minutes, my first reaction was to call Dan. He had been my husband for the last ten years. I called him, and he actually met me at Mercy Hospital where he worked as an ER nurse. Even though I hurt him so much, he always shows up for me when I least expect it. He truly is a good guy; we just were not meant to be married.

As it turned out, I had a concussion so bad that I sounded drunk for two weeks. Thank God I had my mom during this time, or my life would have been worse. She cared for me and the kids. I used to read the same book to Abby every night, and it broke my heart to not be able to do this for her while I was recovering. That was in June.

I felt the pressure of needing money and I went back to work too soon. The bills were not going to pay themselves and Dan had just started paying child support, but I caused so much more damage to my brain by not letting it rest. I was having vision and thinking problems. I still have stuttering issues when I get stressed or work night shift. Sometimes I will say the wrong word when I mean something else because the speech center of my brain was injured. It's hard for me to say the correct thing, even though I know the information.

I was an ICU nurse: people's lives depended on my ability to think and that was not going well. My concussion doctor told me I would never be an ICU nurse again due to the damage, but I refused to believe him. I started therapy at the concussion clinic and got a lawyer. I also started looking for a different job. Then, November 21st came around, and I got a call from my mom saying my best friend was found dead that morning.

LIKE WHAT?

My mom's neighbor was also my best friend. She was like a second mom to my kids. My mom and she shared a yard, so our kids played together all the time. My kids practically lived at my mom's house because of my work schedule. My friend was the only other person I trusted to watch my kids. She was gone just like that. I just could not believe it.

But why? How? What the hell? Why did this happen?

My life was never going to be the same. She was the one person I could tell everything to. I had literally just talked to her the day before. I still have no real reasons for what happened, just my suspicions. I miss her so much. I hope I am making her proud.

Soon after she passed, I was forced to quit my nursing job due to lingering symptoms resulting from the car accident. So, in a matter of months, I lost my job, my best friend, and now was going to lose my house. We had to move because I could not afford the mortgage payment without being a bedside nurse and losing the ability to work extra shifts.

Just a couple months later, in January 2013, I started working as a medical reviewer downtown, and I loved it. It was a way to use my nursing degree and not be bedside. I could not risk hurting a patient. We had to go to court because Dan was still fighting the divorce and filed for full custody of the kids. Abby remembers not wanting to testify against him. The older two did, and Carlyn was given the option to *not* go to his house unless she wanted to.

In March of 2013 the guy I was dating and had left my husband for cheated on me. He emptied the house of all of his things while I was at work one day, including his dogs that my kids, especially Abby, had grown very attached to. I wish I would have understood back then how much my poor life choices were hurting my kids. And I should have known better, because if he could help me cheat and not care, why would he not cheat on me. It was like my life was all red flags of dysfunction. I didn't think of it then, but I deserved it. I felt it was my karma for cheating on my then-soon-to-be ex-husband. Honestly, when I look back, I know that the only reason I survived was by trusting that God would get me through … and he has *big-time*. My mom always told me that life would get better. "Look on the bright side," she would say. She always made me see that it could be worse, and I should be grateful for the blessings I did have. She planted a seed of hope that I have never let go of.

At that moment, though, I was struggling to find a bright side. I was being evicted from our home because the ex-husband would not let me refinance it without him.

Around that same time, I started not being able to swallow food without coughing and choking. I went to the doctor and ordered a sonogram of my thyroid. I then had to get a biopsy. And yes, it was the dreaded word. *Cancer.* I was a single mom still in concussion therapy, still not allowed to work as an ICU nurse, denied disability and trying to appeal, while waiting to find out what I had to do to remove this cancer from my body. This is when I became consciously aware that my healing journey was more than just physical.

Working as a medical reviewer, my office was in downtown Pittsburgh. I had gotten the Audible app so I could have something to listen to on the bus rides home from work. It felt weird to make small talk with strangers every day, so I would listen to books and question all my life choices, wondering how I ended up where I was in life. I wanted to understand why I was the way I was.

You know the old saying, *You can't change what you don't know is broken*?

I did not choose easy fluffy stories to listen to. I listened to books that challenged my whole way of looking at life. I had begun the journey to find the best version of myself by understanding why I did what I did. *The Five Love Languages* by Gary Chapman truly opened my eyes to understand why Dan and I had not worked out. We didn't speak each other's love language! I was very much a *physical touch* and *words of affirmation* person, and Dan was not. I believe he was an *acts of service* person, which is why he always wanted me to clean the house, which I rarely did. Heck, that's even still one of my downfalls. I hate cleaning. I hate living in a dirty house, yet I despise using the vacuum.

My current life situation sucked. If I wanted a different life, I knew I had to change some things. I needed to do something to change it. The one absolute constant in my life since I was little was this sense of protection from God.

I prayed a lot. I had always felt separate from the rest: different, even odd. So, when Dan kept accusing me of having a mental disorder, I thought he could be right. I got a book about borderline personality disorder because Dan had always accused me of being bipolar or borderline. I felt very ashamed. He would always tell me that I was crazy. Tending to your mental health was not a thing to be celebrated as it is today. I started therapy (cognitive behavior therapy) and went twice a week. After discussing my concerns with the professional, I was never diagnosed with anything more than depression.

But shit, I went to the first psychologist and wrote out a timeline of all that had happened to me in the last year, and she asked me, "How haven't you killed yourself yet?"

What? I thought your job was to help me not feel that way? She said most people would have given up by now, and that was just the beginning of my hell year.

I started to exercise again. I started to love being around my kids. I would make dinner and then take Abby and Danny to an elementary school so they could play on the playground while I ran laps around the school. Carlyn would either stay at home, come with us, or be at color guard practice.

I had a small cubicle at work. We were allowed to decorate it a little. I had three Bible quotes printed out and tacked on my boards. I had my kids' pictures like a good mother. But the one thing that got me through every day was Philippians 4:13, "I can do all things through Christ who strengthens me." (NKJV) I still lean into this Bible verse when life gets a little hard to handle.

Until I started looking back to write this book, I didn't even realize that some things were challenges, like going through concussion therapy and having medication changes to alter the chemicals in my brain to help it work better, while being a single mom and working on healing myself. One medication they put me on lowered my blood pressure so much I was passing out. I was so allergic to another one that I couldn't breathe.

At this point in my life, my mom was really my only friend, and she was definitely the only person I trusted to watch my kids. We talked a lot, but she had a gambling addiction that was really running her life. She was so deep into playing the lotto that she even had a bookie. She did not see how it was destroying my dad.

There were secrets I did not know yet.

My mother would blackmail me. She would say that she wouldn't watch the kids so I could go to work unless I paid her. I can recall a specific argument with her: she was telling me she needed gas money, but I had just given her 20 dollars the day before. When asked what she did with it, she said she put it in her tank. I was not stupid. I knew she was only putting a little gas in and buying lotto tickets with the rest.

So, I figured out how many miles it was between our homes, then how much gas her tank could hold, how much gas each mile would use, and how long a tank of gas should last. I showed her the math. She immediately started fighting with me and tried to deflect the conversation to something I did to piss her off. I realized that day that her gambling was a true addiction—she could not understand logic anymore. She was arguing with me the whole time. All she knew was that she needed more money for her lotto tickets. Sadly, addiction runs deep in her side of the family.

As this was going on, I was seeing my doctors about my cancer, and the surgery to remove my thyroid was set for July 6, 2013. Everyone in healthcare knows that new doctors and nurses start in July because of May graduation and then time to pass boards. It's the scariest time to be a patient, and there I was. The tumor had gotten so large in my throat that I could not eat solid food. I was surviving on chocolate covered banana mochas from Sheetz and gooey oatmeal.

Having this surgery was one of the scariest moments in my life because I felt so alone. My mom was not the person I needed her to be, my ex-husband was barely a father, the ex-boyfriend couldn't give two shits less if I made it. He was a real asshole. I hurt my daughter Carlyn the day of my surgery because I wanted Antonio there before I went into surgery so bad that I was spending time desperately calling him while in the waiting room. She was so upset with me and wished I didn't care about him anymore. I did not know how much I was destroying the relationship between me and my oldest daughter then. I didn't think my ex-boyfriend was an asshole then, but hindsight is always 20/20.

I had the surgery at West Penn Hospital in downtown Pittsburgh because that's where the specialist was located. They had to take my parathyroid on the right, so I had to stay a couple days to monitor my calcium levels. On discharge day, no one would come get me. It was pouring down rain, and my dad did not like driving downtown to begin with, let alone in the rain. My mom also refused to drive downtown. I have no siblings to lean on. The pain medication made it so that I do not remember the actual ride home, but I remember it was Dan. My ex-husband drove down, picked me up, and then actually took the kids for a few days so I could recover without having to be a mom at the same time. This is one of the nicer things he ever did for me. He continued to be there for me when I truly needed him to be and still is.

To recap: I lost my best friend (to an overdose), my house, my career as an ICU nurse, and now had my thyroid removed from cancer. I was told I had to have radiation therapy to kill any remaining cancer cells which would be scheduled in a few months after my body healed from the surgery and all the hormonal changes. Mentally, I was so distraught. If I had not started trying to heal mentally and psychologically before that surgery, I do not know where I would be today.

I was still going to therapy twice a week during July and August. I kept listening to different self-help books, which I listed at the back of this book in case you want to read any. I highly recommend *The Five Love Languages*, which I mentioned earlier. It really helped me analyze myself and figure out why my marriage failed … well, besides the toxic abusive relationship that Dan and I created. As a nurse, I was always trying to analyze everything. It's what we are taught to do. Think critically about everything.

I was still mentally unstable from the concussion therapy, and I found out during this time that I am allergic to a lot of medications. They were changing medications every few weeks trying to find something that would help to fix my brain so I could go back to work. Along with that, I was still reeling from the devastation of being told I would never work as an ICU nurse again. It was my heart and soul. I loved having fragile patients and healing them, like the instant gratification in seeing someone's low blood pressure, putting them on Levophed, and watching it come up rapidly. For this self-observed but undiagnosed ADHD nurse, it spoke to me deep in my soul. I knew the doctors did not think I would recover, but I was determined. I kept doing the cognitive exercises and started vestibular therapy. We finally found a medication that worked well, and my life was starting to feel a little more normal.

September came, and the kids were back in school. I was back to work as a medical reviewer, and life seemed to be getting into a rhythm. My mom would come over at 4 a.m. so I could leave for work. I would catch the 5 a.m. bus to downtown, she would get them on the school bus, and then go home.

My mental struggles from the concussion continued, and working as a medical reviewer was not helping my brain heal. I stared at two different computer screens all day, but it was making us enough money to live comfortably.

One day at work, I was talking with my good friend and coworker, Jamie, and she kind of yelled at me. Well, not kind of, she actually yelled at me that I was being a spoiled brat. I was complaining that my mother wasn't going to babysit for me, which I felt entitled to because I had such a shitty childhood—my mother owed me her time. I was an entitled brat, which I realize now. Jamie gave me a different perspective on my mom. She told me that my mother did not in fact owe me anything just because I had a shitty childhood. It was the first time I had ever had someone tell me I needed to be an adult and figure things out myself, without my mother's help.

I then started to look at my mom differently. I had a long talk with Jamie and realized my mom did the best that she could with the information she had and that she really did love me with all of her being. She was only raising me in the best way she knew how. My mom graduated high school and was a stay-at-home mom. She never went to college. She never did anything to advance her career. In fact, she lived to make me happy.

My mother was 19 when she met my dad. He was her only boyfriend and became her husband for 37 years until her death. She loved being a mom and a grandma. I never appreciated her while she was alive; well, I did for about a week.

After Jamie and I had this conversation (which continued on the bus ride home), I was driving home from the park and ride area, and a song came on the radio about God hearing our prayers. I lost it. I was bawling and screaming at God. I was pouring my heart out and asking him why I had to suffer so much. I only listened to K-Love, which is a Christian radio station, after being challenged by a coworker in 2011 while in the middle of a very nasty divorce. We had been listening to K-Love while working on the ambulance one day, and he challenged me to listen to it for 30 days and see if my life changed. My life did not change, but my perspective did, so I kept listening to it and still do to this day.

I love God. I didn't mean to be disrespectful by screaming at him, but I was at one of the lowest points in my life. I was a single mom, feeling all alone and had just been through surgery to remove cancer a few months before. I was struggling with the concussion therapy and the hormonal changes that come from not having a thyroid anymore. I was battling with my ex-husband about everything. He was paying child support, but it was not much, so I was pretty much the sole provider for my three children. I did not want them to suffer, so I would forgo things for myself to ensure they had what they wanted; yet, some of the hardest days were still to come.

When I was trying to heal from the concussion in 2013, I had pushed myself so hard. I was going to the park and running or taking the kids to the school and running around the school while they played in the playground. I pushed through all the time despite having major migraines that would cause me to be bedridden for hours. I refused to give up. I kept Philippians 4:13 close to my heart.

My conversation with Jamie happened on a Monday or Tuesday, and I had asked my mom to watch Abby for me on Friday because the older two had a football game on Friday night and a band competition on Saturday. Abby did not like sitting through their activities, so I dropped the older two off at the high school, and Abby and I went to Grandma's house. I spent some time there hanging out with my parents Friday night before going back to pick up the older kids. I remember this conversation like it was yesterday. My mom was talking about her brother needing to have his foot removed due to diabetes complications. I told her, "You better hope you go first because I can take care of Daddy, but you and I will kill each other." I said it half joking, not knowing it would be one of the last conversations I would have with my mother. Sadly, our relationship was very hostile and toxic at this point. I kissed Abby and left to pick up the other two.

On Saturday morning, I dropped Carlyn and Danny off at the high school and went to get coffee and doughnuts. Then I headed to my parents' house. I asked my mom if I could talk to her alone. We sat on her front porch swing, and I said, "Mom, I love you. I know you never meant to hurt me as a child, and you were doing the best you could with the information you had at the time. I recognize that your parents were abusive and strict, and you went in the opposite direction in raising me, thinking it had to be the better option. I do not feel it was right, but I know you did not do it to intentionally hurt me."

She responded with "I didn't."

I knew it wasn't going to be an easy conversation, but I had to let her know that while I did not agree with how she raised me, I know she did her best.

We agreed to disagree and try to repair our mother-daughter bond. That was Saturday, September 21, 2013. We went to church together with the kids the next day, and everything was going great in my life for about 24 hours. Monday, Carlyn took off from school so we could go dress shopping for homecoming because we had gone to all the usual places, and she did not like anything. I had to hide money from my mom at this point because she was still blackmailing me. So, we did not tell her that Carlyn had found a dress, but it was four hundred dollars. My mom would not babysit unless I gave her money. (It wasn't until her death that my father and I realized how bad her gambling addiction was.)

Monday night, my ex-husband called and said he was throwing out the bunk beds that my mom had given him when I kicked him out. She always told me she liked him better than me. My mom said I had to give her money for gas if I wanted her to go get the bunk beds. I told her I did not have any because I knew I needed it for Carlyn's homecoming dress. My mom was so mad at me that she was screaming.

When she called me at 4 a.m. the next morning to say she wasn't feeling well, I told her, "Don't worry about it. I'm staying home. You feel better and call me if you need anything." Those were the last words I ever spoke to my mom. The next phone call came from my dad, saying that he was taking her to the ER at McKeesport Hospital because her blood sugar machine was reading high, and she had been throwing up for the last few hours.

Now, she was an obese woman with diabetes who never took care of herself. She lived for me and her grandchildren. She had breast cancer at age 47 in her left breast and had months of radiation and several doses of chemo. All of that took a toll on her heart and it was catching up with her. This day happened to be ten years after all of that.

So, when she called me to say she hoped I wasn't going to work because she couldn't watch the kids, I figured she was still pissed at me from the night before when I refused to give her money. I have played this day over in my head probably a thousand times. Abby had stayed home that day, and we were on our way to the bus stop to pick up Carlyn when my phone rang. It was Aunt Barb, my mom's sister, calling. She said, "Your mom is being flown to Shadyside Hospital. She had a heart attack."

My mind was racing. I was so mad at myself at that moment.
Why didn't I go check on her today?
Why did they wait so long to take her to the hospital?
What am I going to do?
How is this happening?

I very quickly made a phone call to Danny's friend's dad. He was his scoutmaster for Boy Scouts and a neighbor who only lived down the road. We dropped Abby off there, and they went to get Danny for me. Carlyn and I flew, and I mean I have no idea what speed I was driving, I just knew that we made it to McKeesport Hospital before STAT MedEvac got there.

We were taken to the cath lab waiting room where my dad was sitting alone. He did not quite realize the severity of the situation. I did. I knew the odds were not in her favor, given her medical history. I was able to see her in the cath lab. She was intubated and lifeless. The gurney went past us as she was leaving with STAT MedEvac to be flown to the higher-level-of-care hospital on the other side of the city. They let us give her kisses before they took her. I had previously worked with two of the nurses who coded my mom. I will never forget how amazing Melissa and Patrick were. Melissa was kind enough to tell me how bad it was, to give me the results of her blood gases and labs, and I knew the outcome. Post-arrest patients rarely survive.

In that moment, I knew my life was forever changed. I heard once on the radio that life is 10% what happens to us and 90% how we react to it.

I thought my mom had the stomach flu and only figured out she wasn't feeling well because she was having a heart attack after the fact. And for years I beat myself up because *I should have saved her.* I was an ICU nurse! How could I miss this? How did I not go to her house and assess her earlier in the day? I have been trying to forgive myself for fighting with her that night. I know logically it is not my fault she had the heart attack, but emotionally and as a child of a parent with an addiction, I wanted more time to fix the relationship.

I drove my dad and Carlyn to Shadyside, and we met my aunt and uncle there. That was a pretty scary drive. I was grateful that I had been taking the busway to work in Pittsburgh a few months back and knew that a car can drive on the busway with its flashers on. Wanna guess how we got to Shadyside so quickly? You guessed it. I didn't care if anyone called the cops. My mom was dying, and I surely was not sitting in Pittsburgh traffic at three o'clock in the afternoon.

I have had to learn how to make the most of this life.

We spent the next four days with the ups and downs of the intensive care unit: being transferred from Shadyside after getting an ECMO (aka life support)—catheter placed and being put on the heart transplant list. There was a moment I had with my mom as she was being wheeled out of the ambulance at Presbyterian

Hospital from Shadyside. She grabbed my hand and she squeezed when I said, "I love you." She was still in there. I had hope for a day or so that she might be able to recover from this. I wanted so desperately for her to be OK. Then, she started having strokes from blood clots caused by the machines that were keeping her alive.

I truly believe that everything happens for a reason. I remember kneeling on my floor at my bed, bawling and begging, *God why?* Screaming at him not to take her. The cardiothoracic surgeon told me she needed a transplant or she would die, but she could not get stable enough to even be evaluated for a transplant. I thought, *That's it. I will not let her suffer.*

I have seen too many families hold out that last drop of hope, begging for a miracle while their loved one is being tortured, uncomfortable, and in pain—always being poked and prodded. I was not going to let my mother suffer. She was going to lose her leg from the ECMO machine they used trying to save her. She was having little strokes as clots were being thrown into her brain from the machine. She was on a blood thinning medication, but it was not working.

As a nurse, I knew she would never have the life that she had known before this. The recovery would have been too much. She would not have healed correctly because she was a diabetic. She would have been in a nursing home if she even survived and made it to a transplant. I could not let that happen to her. We choose to make her comfortable. This was one of the hardest days of my life.

She lasted for a few hellish days in the hospital, only to succumb to her illness on October 1, 2013. My ex-husband surprised me and was there for his children the day my mother died. He even came to the funeral. He could have left his mother and her husband at home, though.

Being a nurse and knowing what was happening to my mom made her last few days some of the worst of my life. It was so hard to hold onto hope as she lay there on a ventilator, knowing her medical history and knowing that surviving a hospital cardiac arrest was so slim. It shook me to my nursing core. I knew it was going to be a while before I could go back to an ICU as a staff nurse. Thank the Lord that my mom had talked me into going for disability and filing all the paperwork before she passed because having that time off to help my dad and my kids was priceless to me. "Everything always happens for a reason," she would say. My mom would tell me to always look for the reason and that things happened *for* us not *to* us.

On October 1, 2013, I became a motherless daughter. She became my angel. As I write this, I realize it's been ten years. I never would have believed it, but this healing journey of mine—this life-changing, gut-wrenching event that took me away from nursing for longer than I expected—has actually helped me be a better nurse.

I have used my pain to help hundreds of families deal with the decision to let go of their loved ones because I can say, "I truly know your pain. I have had to do this with my mother, and it sucks." And my patients' families know that I speak from the heart.

Losing my mother has left a hole in my heart and in our family. You do learn to live again. It is just different. My mom was the glue that held her family together. My aunt Barb, my mom's sister, did not speak to me for years before my mom died, but after, she told me I killed my mom. I screamed at her. I tried to explain how bad the situation was, but she had no medical knowledge and did not understand. I tried to help her understand that it would have taken Jesus himself to come and heal my mother. But in hindsight, my mom was not meant to be here anymore. She had a more important job now. It was to be our angel. To help line up all the amazing things God had in store for our lives.

Just a month later, I became the patient.

In November, I had to receive radiation and was not allowed to be around my kids for weeks. I spent that time really trying to heal from the year of loss after loss after loss. I used this time of despair to figure out who I was as a person. I spent many days on my knees praying. I became a prayer warrior for others. I would get emails for prayer requests, because while I could not change what had happened to me over the last 12 months, I wanted to do something to help someone else. I found out that I had a direct line to God. I would call them "instaprayers" because it seemed almost instantaneously that I would get answers. I didn't realize it then, but now I do.

One of my prayers, written as a note to God, was asking him for a man who would love me fully. I wrote out all the things I wanted him to be and how I wanted him to look. I had no idea that our moms would meet in heaven and make the arrangements.

In life, there are moments meant to break you; it is in that brokenness that you find your inner strength. I found mine from June 2012 to December 2013. This time was meant to tear me down and strip me of everything I thought I was … and it did. It ripped away so much of my ego, my false sense of security, and my beliefs of who I thought I was. I was stripped of everything I held dear to my heart and about who I was as a human. But this was all necessary to rebuild me into the woman I am today.

I was very blessed to have already been in therapy—seeing a cognitive behavioral therapist—and working on myself when my mom died. The loss of my mother forced me to be a more involved mom. I had relied on her to care for my children while I worked and built my career, and in an instant, my life changed.

The ramifications of her death were deep for all of us. My father had never written a check in his life. He had never gone to the grocery store and bought food. He had never cooked a meal for himself … well, maybe 30 years ago but not recently. My mother was everything for him. I watched her give up so many things for me and my kids to have whatever we wanted in life. My kids were privileged to have such a giving woman as their grandma, but sadly, that was all gone. Carlyn was 15, Danny was 13, and Abby was eight years old at the time of her death. Abby has now lived more of her life without her grandma than she had years with her.

The pain of grief lingered in our home for years. Sadly, I truly believe that if my mom were still alive, I would have a relationship with my oldest daughter, Carlyn. When my mom died, Carlyn lost the main mother figure in her life because they were together so much due to my work schedule, which included extra days I chose to work. We didn't get to have the same mother-daughter bond that she had forged with her grandmother. The two of us seemed more like friends, and it's easier to walk away from a friend you're pissed at.

While I was tucked away due to the radiation treatments and not allowed to interact with my family, I started trying to find ways to have a better life. To spend less time working and more time with my children. During this time, I had heard about setting intentions and wrote in a note on my phone the type of man I wanted to be with forever. I put it out there and then actually forgot about it— went on with my daily life.

I was learning to love me. I was still going to cognitive behavioral therapy once a week to learn to regulate my emotions. I listened to the book *Emotional Intelligence* by Daniel Goleman to become a better person and a better mom. I read the *4-Hour Work Week* by Tim Ferriss and realized I wanted more out of life and that happiness was a matter of perspective. I decided that my happiness comes from the love of God and his belief in me.

During this time, I was not very emotionally available for my kids, but I did not know that then. All I knew was survival mode. I was doing whatever I had to do to pay the bills and make sure my kids had food and clothing. I felt like life kept kicking me.

Dealing with loss is a universal human experience: loss of a marriage, loss of a career, loss of a family, and loss of a parent. Each of these gives life perspective. I started listening to Abraham Hicks and learning how she describes life. She describes life in contrast. All of the loss is here so we can enjoy the good times. It is how we deal with the loss that defines us. I refused in that moment to wallow. I had to be strong. I now had to help my dad learn how to be an adult. I had to figure out what I was going to do about ever going back to work and how that was going to work itself out. I should have been depressed. I was not. I leaned into my Bible. I leaned into prayer. I continued to be a prayer warrior for others. I prayed so much in the next year for other people that it became a way of life for me. I know others saw Jesus through me because I allowed myself to be a vessel of love.

Chapter 5
The Year After My Mom Left Us

"To accomplish much, you must first lose everything."[8]
~ Ernesto che Guevara

2014

The year after my mother died was and still is sort of a blur. The month after her death, I was still in shock. I was told I had to have radiation to completely remove the cancer from my throat. So there I was a single mom, with no siblings to help, and I couldn't be around my kids for a month. God knew I needed help and sent an old flame to reach out. Jason was an old boyfriend from high school who I ran into at Target one night, and we reconnected. He was someone I never stopped caring about. He explained that he was living at his mother's house just a few minutes away from me. I really was not in a head space to have a new boyfriend, but he wasn't new; he was recycled. Back then I had no idea what it was doing to my daughters to see me so needy and graspy for love and attention from a man. I still had no understanding of self-love at this point.

We had a few dates, he met my kids, and he stayed over a couple times. Then one day he just didn't leave. Now, the good thing was that he was a Navy veteran who worked on a nuclear submarine, so he could be exposed to my radiation without any effects, and he was loving enough to make meals for my kids. Jason took me back and forth to my radiation treatments. He helped me plan a birthday party for my mom in her honor, and I

---

[8] https://quotefancy.com/quote/1047493/Ernesto-Che-Guevara-To-accomplish-much-you-must-first-lose-everything

loved his family. He pretty much cooked Thanksgiving dinner since I was not allowed to touch other people's food yet. He helped me get unpacked in my new place and organize my life a little.

Some back story: When we were dating in high school, I had gone with his family to see him graduate from the Navy. His mom always thought he and I were meant to be together, and she helped make that first Christmas without my mom a little easier. She had me bring my dad to her place for Christmas dinner.

I am so thankful for all the help he and his family gave me when I was down and out and had nowhere to turn. His mother showed me so much love; I can never repay her. I was going to my concussion therapy but still not working. Jason helped me with all the med changes and multiple different allergic reactions. They put me on a medication called a beta blocker to help with the constant migraines, and it dropped my blood pressure so low I was passing out—that one did not work. I constantly felt like I was being stabbed in the head and could not focus. The stress of my life was causing severe abdominal pain from the Crohn's exacerbations. I was mentally distraught pretty much every day.

I knew I could not change my situation, but I thought maybe praying every day for other people instead of wallowing in my own self-pity would change my life. And it did. I prayed for hours each day. I signed up to receive random strangers' emails requesting prayers. I don't even remember what I prayed for for those people, but I know it gave me such a connection with my higher self, my God, and the universe. It sparked a change in me. It gave me back a sense of purpose. When my concussion doctor told me I would never be an ICU nurse again, I was so lost, but being stuck in a room alone for weeks while going through radiation, I found myself.

Despite the grief, I felt a sense of purpose at the beginning of 2014. I still wasn't sure what that purpose was yet, but I knew I was to survive for something greater than myself. It was the same sense I had felt when I started nursing school. It was a deep knowing that I was created to do so much more than just pay my bills and die.

I know that, as a nurse, you felt a sense of purpose or you would not have stuck with nursing. This is a difficult field to work in. I have gotten punched, kicked, spit on, spit at, and had a bedside table chucked at me. We get verbally abused by patients, their families, and even doctors sometimes.

But it's that one patient whose life you know you made a difference in, who pushes you to carry on. It's the one *thank you* from a distraught family member who sends in a card and snacks with your name singled out that touches your soul and helps you want to come back and do it again. But my soul was so broken from all I had been through that my purpose was wavering.

In early 2014, I realized that I was *my one patient*. I was the one who needed my love and support. I started to love myself. I started to put myself first in life, and that's when things started to change. I started walking and just spending time with my kids and really loving my life right where I was. I continued reading self-help books to grow and become better.

We moved again in April 2014, and this time, I left Jason behind … or he left himself. Either way, it was the right choice. It was just me, my kids, and my dad. That was my family.

I was still in therapy once a week, but I started to feel like I could function as a human again. I had a few setbacks during my healing, of course. If you have ever had anything to heal from, you know the journey is ups and downs and breakdowns and breakthroughs. I was hospitalized a few times for Crohn's exacerbations, where I needed a few days of IV antibiotics and CT scans. On the last one, my doctor wanted to try new therapies, so I started getting prepped for those—the TB tests and all the vaccines. But when I went to see the gastroenterologist he said, "You had thyroid cancer. You can't have the immunologics." So, back to square one.

He suggested I get a resection done. So here I was again, two years in a row, heading into surgery in July. When I say I was mentally tested on every level, I truly was. The prep for colon surgery was no real solid food for a month. I could only ingest the protein shakes that the doctor ordered for me. Then clears for the week before. I was willing to do anything to prevent sepsis. As I was drinking one of the shakes one morning, I kept smelling it. It had a very familiar smell. My oldest daughter was looking at me funny and asked what I was doing. I couldn't figure it out, but it smelled so familiar. It didn't taste bad, just like a protein shake. Then all of a sudden it hit me like a ton of bricks. I yelled it out so loud I think I startled Carlyn.

"TUBE FEEDS! HE GAVE ME TUBE FEEDS!"

It was a cruel turn of events for this ICU nurse. I had hung these on so many patients I never thought I would be drinking them. UGH. I started to crack up. My teenager didn't get the irony, but I'm sure you do.

The surgery went well. I had dropped so much weight in that month by only consuming tube feeds in a box that I felt pretty even though my stomach had just gotten cut open and rearranged. Mentally, I was in such a good space. Now, I had my health and my kids, and I was really looking forward to a new life of being single. I had started to apply to jobs outside of being a nurse. I had applied to be an insurance agent and, once, a medical device salesperson. I was still going to concussion therapy and behavioral therapy. I had to get special glasses because of the concussion, so I could stare at a computer and not get a migraine. I had started going to church again.

The kids were going to start school soon, but there was one thing I needed to do.

My dad belonged to the Vietnam Veterans Motorcycle Club (VNV MC) for over 30 years. This was a huge part of why I am the way that I am. That's how I learned that family is more than just your blood relatives. So this club has a huge blow out party once a year to celebrate. That party has always been the week before school starts. I am talking about thousands of people from all over who would come to this party. We didn't have a lot of money at the time, and I had been trying to fix my dad's life since my mom passed. We found out she was floating checks with her sister so they could gamble, and she had a secret bank account. But I had promised my dad that I would find a way to get him to this party.

It was the Wednesday before the party, and I dropped off the kids to my ex-husband. I packed the car, and we left for the campground. It was about a three-hour car ride. The last time I attended one of these parties, Carlyn was about six months old; she was now going to be a junior in high school. When I last attended, I had won the bike game called the Wienie Bite. It is a motorcycle game where the guy drives and the girl rides on the back and is driven under a structure that has a hotdog dipped in mustard hanging from a string. The goal of this game is to bite off as much of the hotdog as possible while the driver goes under but does not put his feet down. If he puts his feet down, you are disqualified. I felt I had a reputation to uphold. I needed to play and win again. I spent Wednesday evening, Thursday, and Friday morning trying to find someone to drive me in this contest. The competition was Saturday.

On Friday evening, it was still light out a couple hours before sunset, and I had still not found anyone to be my driver. I was sitting around the campfire with my honorary aunts, Joyce and Ginny, and I spotted this hunk walking across the field toward our camp. I leaned over to Joyce and whispered, "Who's that hot guy?"

Now remember, I had no intention of finding a guy, I did not want a guy in my life. I was so happy being single. I was working on myself. The last thing I wanted in my life right now was a boyfriend. Fuck that.

Joyce replied, "That's Little Bob."

"Oh,"

"He's one of the guys in W Chapter Second Brigade."

"Do you know if he rode up?"

"Yeah, that's his bike."

It was a Harley Ultra parked directly in front of our campsite. It was the type of bike I knew I needed because it had handles for the backseat passenger so I could stick my feet in them and have more balance for the game.

As he and his dad walked over to the camp, they were talking to one of the guys. I went marching up to him with such an attitude in my short shorts and tank top. I walked over like I owned the place.

I said to the sexiest biker I had ever seen, "You got a girlfriend? 'cause I ain't stepping on anybody's toes."

"No."

"You have a bike here?" I already knew the answer.

"Yeah."

"You feel like driving me in the Wienie Bite contest tomorrow?"

"Sure."

"Great, thanks."

And I turned around and walked back over to the campfire. I was so pleased with myself.

A few hours went by, and people came and went. We all ate dinner, and it was late now. The band was starting to play at the pavilion. You could hear the music from our campsite. Little Bob's nickname is quite deceiving. It's kind of like Little John from Robin Hood. He is so tall. Come to find out he is six foot four inches. I am only five foot four inches.

He ended up hanging out with us around the campfire all night. He and I had so much fun. I jokingly (but not so jokingly) told him I had a dowry, but instead of him being paid to take me, he would have to pay three hundred thousand in cash, if he wanted to date me. I said I had no intentions of meeting a guy. I was there to make sure my dad did not miss this party just because my mom was gone.

Bob had told me that he always liked my mom and how kind she was. Which I knew. She would make breakfast for like 30 people and then feed all the single guys as good karma, so when my dad would go places without her, she knew someone would feed him.

Finally, around 5 a.m., I decided I needed to get some sleep, and Bob walked me over to my dad's camper. He leaned in, and we kissed. It was the most magical kiss I had ever had. I swear I saw fireworks in the sky at that moment. Maybe it was the entire bottle of wine—the big gallon one—I had drank. I don't know. It was as if my soul found the missing half it had been searching for all its life. It was so tender and amazing. My life changed in that instant. He went to his tent, and I went to sleep.

I slept for a couple hours, and then got up and made sure we were signed up for the Wienie Bite contest. I made sure Bob was awake and OK. We did just stay up all hours of the night drinking and bullshitting around the campfire.

The contest was around 11 a.m.

Lori Ann Lewicki

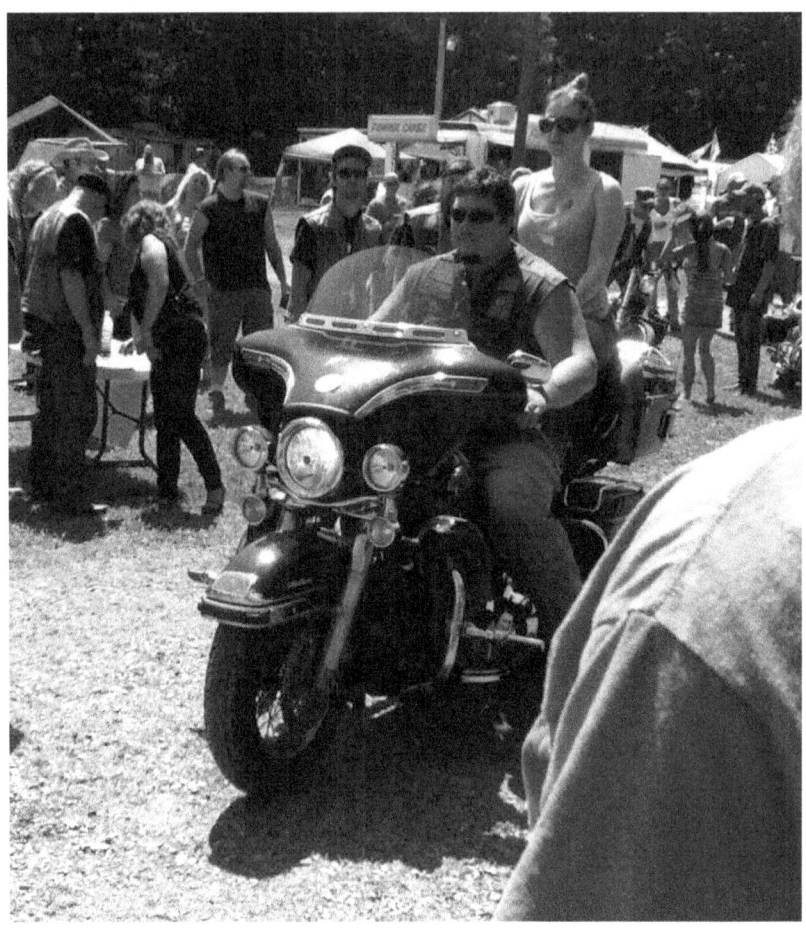

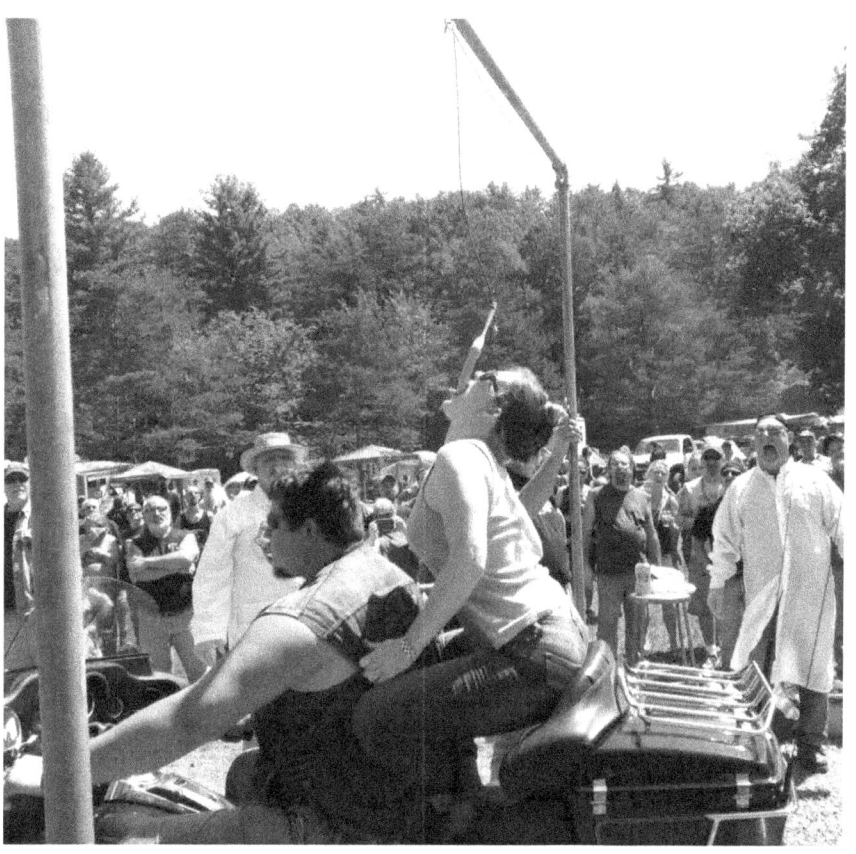

Lori Ann Lewicki

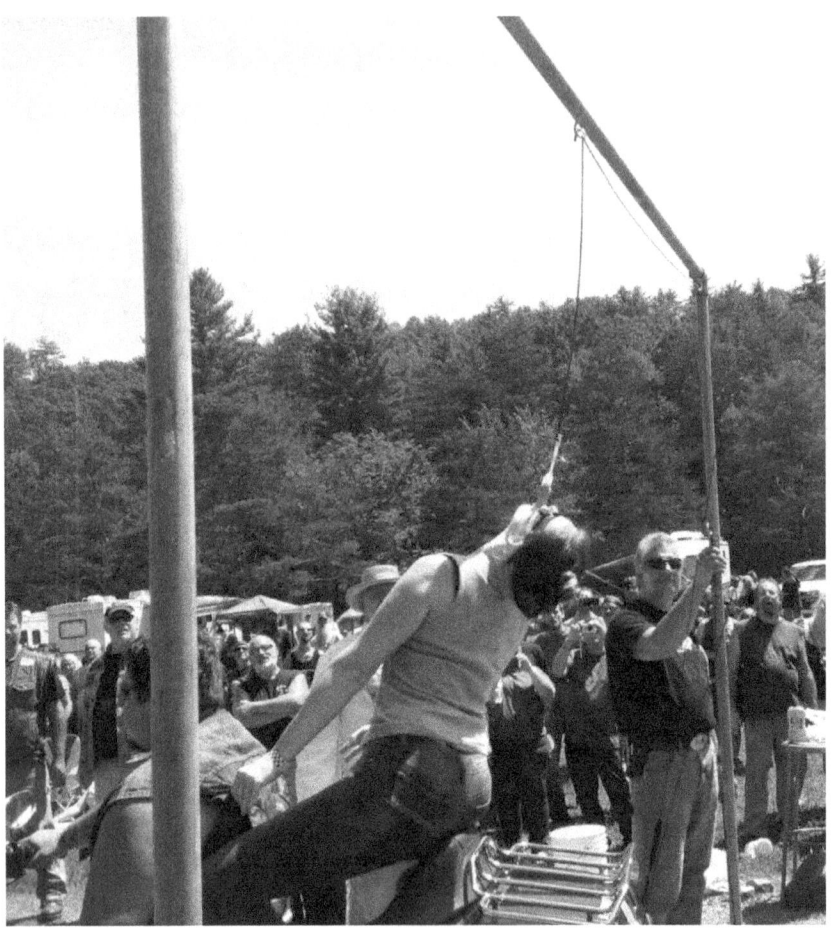

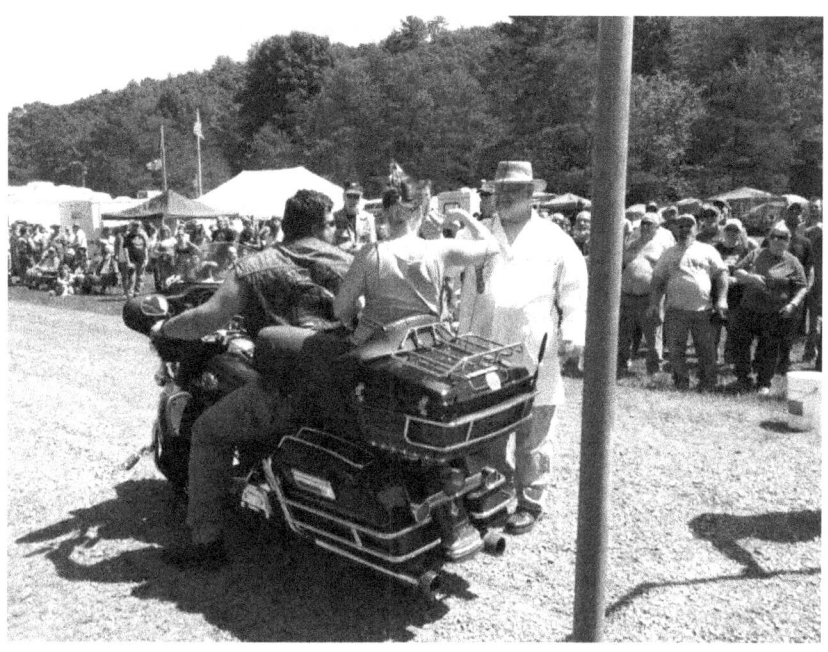

I did not win the contest that day, but it's OK. I won at life. Bob promised to take me for a real bike ride after his chapter meeting. They have a meeting once a month, and since they were all there for the party, they just had the meeting there. He drove me over to my camp, and I got a shower while I waited for him. I still did not think much of anything would come from my time with him. I was still not looking for any serious relationship. I was just there to have a good time.

It was the bike ride that had me weak at the knees. He took me on a four-hour ride all over the countryside of Pennsylvania. It was the best first date I had ever had. The best part for me was when we stopped for gas at a Sheetz, and I hopped off the bike like we had been married for years and stuck my hand out for money because I wanted a drink. He handed me money and never said a word. We rode for a little longer and then headed back to camp. I fell in love on that ride. I leaned in, and he smelled like comfort. I just knew I would always be protected. I still was not sure where this would go long-term, but for the moment, I was so happy. I truly did not know—and told myself I didn't care—if I ever heard from him again. I knew there was something special, but I wasn't going to let myself fall for anyone. I had a wall up. We hung out Saturday night, but then he had to go work security for the band, and I went back to my campsite.

Sunday morning, we exchanged numbers, but honestly I never thought he was going to call me. I just wanted to make sure he made it home safely. I am that friend. I expect texts after a night out, so I know that you made it home safe.

When my phone rang five hours later, it was Bob. I was so excited and scared at the same time. Despite all the shit I had swam through, I still held out hope for a knight in shining armor. I always dreamed of the fairytale love I saw with my parents: my dad adored my mom. He still talks about how she was the love of his life. I had one friend, Vince, who made fun of me all the time for still wanting a romance after the shit Antonio put me through. But here it was. I did not remember it when I met Bob, but I had written a list in my notes on my phone of the perfect guy for me when Antonio broke my heart a year before.

Over the months of talking with Bob and dating him, I realized he checked off the entire list except his hair color. I had written I wanted a redhead because I always had a thing for redheads. This was an exercise of manifesting before I knew what manifesting was. But it was not all roses. My oldest daughter was so pissed at me for "going after another guy." She refused to get to know Bob and hated him before she ever knew him because I had promised no more guys. No matter how much I knew this was different, it did not matter. When Bob and I started dating, it was the beginning of the dissolution of my relationship with my daughter, but I figured she would come around.

I did not know there were other forces working against me to destroy my relationship with Carlyn. It goes back to the blending of families. My ex-husband had remarried and his new wife was texting Carlyn and telling her not to respect me. She told her what to say to make me cry and how to hurt me. One day when Carlyn was at a color guard competition, Abby found her other phone that had all of these texts from the new wife to Carlyn saying all kinds of nasty things about me. I lost the relationship with my daughter over the next year. It was her senior year of high school. It was supposed to be filled with so much love. She had all the emails for her color guard squad sent to her and didn't tell me about things the parents were doing to honor them. I felt horrible that I was not given the chance to show her she mattered to me, but in her defense, she knew we did not have extra money to participate. It was a hard time for all of us, and we each processed it so differently. I understand now that it was just what needed to happen, so that I could make this healing journey.

She slowly kept pushing me out of her life, and I knew I still had so much growing and changing I needed to do. We were constantly fighting and screaming till, one day, she blew up. She was only supposed to go to her friend's house for a couple days, but she never returned home. It has been eight years. I tried for years to have a relationship with her, but she has requested that I not be in her life. I had gotten a life coach that was helping me process these emotions, and once I learned about boundaries, I had to respect hers. My coach taught me that if I kept trying to force my way into her life, I would push her out forever. I still love her with all my heart, and I pray and hope that someday I will be part of her life. So, I had to let her go and live her life. I pray for her all the time. I am going to hold on to hope because it has gotten me through all these years. God has always been faithful to me. Philippians 4:13, "I can do all things through Christ who strengthens me." That verse continues to be my mantra.

What gets you through the hard days? Do you pray? Meditate? Exercise? Listen to music? Try some of the techniques I share in this book and see if they help, like shifting your mindset, writing down what you want out of life, going to therapy. I continue to share what helped me in the chapters that follow.

Chapter 6
Learning from Great Thinkers

"Those who seek a better life must first become a better person."[9]
~ Jim Rohn

Carlyn moving out before her senior year was complete was my lowest point. She called me a "pill head" because of all the meds I was on from the concussion therapy. They had me on uppers to stay awake and downers to go to sleep. I was popping pills constantly, albeit prescribed, but it didn't matter. I was so broken. She was my best friend, but I had not been a mother to her, and since my mom's death, Carlyn and I never did figure out how to have a mother-daughter relationship. I thank God for sending me Bob and giving me hope in love because he held me at my lowest and helped me grow and change. He is always right beside me, supporting me in every endeavor. I was so upset, and a cousin reached out to me and suggested I watch the movie *The Secret*. It opened my eyes to the Law of Attraction (basically, what you focus on, you bring into your life) and manifesting, and I have not looked back.

Part of my major healing came when I joined Amway (an independent health and beauty company), which is a cool story of meeting my best friend. I was taking a break from being a bedside nurse because I was still healing from the concussion therapy and what all the medication changes did to me. I had tried to go back to working as an ICU nurse, and it was very traumatic because I was still processing my mother's death. I tried being a nurse manager for a few months and realized that I was too honest. I stood up to

---

[9] https://quotefancy.com/quote/838213/Jim-Rohn-Those-who-seek-a-better-life-must-first-become-a-better-person

management and protected my nurses, so that position did not last long. They wanted a *yes* person, and I could not fit that role. At that point, I said I was done with being treated like crap and wanted to do something to help others have a better life, not just fix them or try to after the damage was done.

I started working at LA Fitness, a local gym, to help people be healthier before they are broken, before they end up needing a nurse. As a nurse, I repaired the broken, and I was not sure I ever wanted to work as a nurse again. I loved the concept of helping others be healthy and preventing illness, not just putting a Band-Aid on the problem like I feel our current healthcare system does. I wanted to help others reach their true potential of wellness.

In my own life, I started to put myself first and get my life healthy and really wanted to make a difference for others, so when a woman was at the gym advertising for a chiropractor she worked for, I started chatting with her. I told her I had a migraine, she gave me vitamin water, and my headache was gone for the first time in months. I was amazed. We talked a little bit and decided to meet again in a couple days. We ended up meeting on my mom's birthday, December 20th, and we just clicked. I loved her energy and wanted to do whatever she was doing. Michelea introduced me to Amway and a whole new way to view the world.

Because of Amway, Bob and I started reading and listening to books by the great thinkers of the world like Zig Zigler, Andrew Carnegie, Napoleon Hill, and Charles Haanel. I was learning concepts of mind-hacking and hardwiring your brain for happiness. I was encouraged like I had never been. I was told I was awesome at Amway's business meetings, and I started to really thrive. My kids noticed the positive changes. Bob and I became Amway distributors in January of 2016. We had also just gotten married in October of 2015, so we had a lot of stressors. I know 100% that being in Amway and around so many positive people saved my life. Plus, Amway's products saved my life. I loved getting paid to buy products that I was already buying like shampoo and laundry detergent, but the supplements helped me get off all the meds from the concussion clinic and helped me be the healthiest I had ever been. I don't even want to think about what my life would be like if I had not been around those people and had not been introduced to a new way of thinking and living. I definitely wouldn't be the person I am today.

One of the biggest life lessons I learned from the self-help books was that I cannot change the past, but if I want a great future, I need to let go of the anger and the hurt. I have mentioned that my oldest daughter hasn't really spoken to me in a few years, but I still do not blame her. I know she had a rough childhood. I was always working when she was little and when she was a teenager I was going through so much of my own shit that I forgot I needed to be a mom first. I have so much regret from losing our relationship. But, being in Amway and around so many positive, forward-thinking individuals made me want to be a better person.

When Carlyn was growing up, she saw me try to drink away my problems. She was there for all the fights with my ex-husband. She testified in court during the custody battle. My desire to be the mom she always wanted and needed made me change. It was her birth all those years ago that showed me what love meant, but it was Jim Rohn's teachings that helped me forgive myself for not being the mother my kids deserved. Carlyn had already moved out and never got to see how I had changed, though. She has no idea how much she has made my life better just by being my daughter. Each of my children have had such a positive impact on the woman I am today. Danny always finds a way to make me smile when I am stressed out. He has chosen to be a part of my life through all the challenges and now enjoys all the benefits of me trying to make it up to him for all the mistakes I made years ago. Abby told me I give her hope in humans because she watched me grow and learn and change, proving that I am different now.

It wasn't an overnight change. It has been a slow and steady improvement. I've had many good days, but I still have my bad days where I am not on top of my game. I am not perfect and never claimed to be. (Spoiler alert: neither are you. Nobody is.) I started changing my inner self-talk first. I no longer told myself I was *dumb*. When I realized I got this behavior from my dad, it stung. I heard him call himself *stupid* for something, and it hurt. I started to recognize that I got my negativity from my dad. He still calls himself *stupid* when he forgets things, which is really bad now that he has dementia.

A few years ago, I tried to teach him about energy. The nice part about him going through radiation therapy for prostate cancer was that it gave us a lot of time together. I used some of that time to teach him positive self-talk, as I drove him to treatments and doctors' appointments. This is why I believe everything happens for a reason: if I didn't have the concussion and wasn't trying to get disability, I would not have been off work and able to be there for my dad when he needed me. He did well, being kind and using positive self-talk for a few years, but the dementia has stolen that and he is back to being a dick, acting like he did when I was a child. Thankfully, I have learned how to emotionally protect myself in a way I did not know when I was younger.

I have read dozens of self-empowerment books, and I want to share some of them with you. So, I have provided a list of books in the appendix, if you want the information firsthand. One of my favorite books that changed my life was Mel Robbins' *The Five Second Rule.* She was having crippling anxiety and noticed her children were starting to follow in her footsteps. So she developed a trick to make her mind stop going down the anxiety black hole and decrease the panic. The trick is to have a happy place in mind. For me, that is a certain creek—not *shit creek!*—within an hour of my home (you'll recognize it as the cover photo) that I can get to relatively easily. I have spent hours in this creek, meditating and filling my cup. So, this is the happy thought, the next part is, when you feel the anxiety starting to kick in, you say *5,4,3,2,1* and insert that happy thought

One time, in particular, we were heading to Washington, D.C., for an Amway conference. It was raining pretty heavily, and it was dark after 9 p.m. It was "country dark," meaning there were no streetlights to light the way. I was driving because being a passenger was causing me too much anxiety, but also *driving in these conditions* was increasing my anxiety, causing it to rear its head. My husband reminded me of the technique, and I kept repeating out loud *5,4,3,2,1* and thinking my happy thought. I kept doing this trick over and over again until I started to feel better. Bob was actually the one who read this book by Mel Robbins first—in a way, to help me—and then asked me to read it. He really is my better half. We complement each other so perfectly. Together, we have shifted so many little things over the years. It was not this huge one-time thing. But first, I had to have the desire to constantly be better than the version of myself from the day before. I have shared this method so many times with patients over the years to help them.

The more I learn about mindset and energy frequencies, the more I understand why this works. Energy cannot be created or destroyed. We are made of energy and all of our feelings have different frequency levels. The anxiety I was having was causing my frequency to be more on the lower end of the spectrum; now, I set intentions about my day to have a higher frequency, meaning I operate with a more positive outlook. I do what is called "bubble protection," which I learned from a mind-over-medicine book. Before work every day, I say a prayer, asking God to put a bubble around me to protect me and my energy. I ask him to wrap the bubble in pink love so anything that bumps into it bounces back to the person with love. This comes in handy when the nurses I am working with are exceptionally cranky. It also helps when the stories of the patients are extremely sad. I found, as a nurse, I was taking on a lot of pain from my patients. My patients were not physically hurting me, but the circumstances that lead them to be patients were sad. I believe most nurses are empaths and have an ability to feel other people's emotions, which is why we get so burned out. I do not have any scientific proof of this, but I consider my exhaustion after a day of work that is especially emotionally draining to be evidence enough.

You know that little glimmer in your gut we call your "nurse's intuition"? Yes that. That is your internal navigation system. Everyone has one, but not everyone listens to it. Did you ever have a patient that just did not look right? His or her vital signs did not specifically show any signs of distress, but you just felt there was something wrong? *Yes!* That is your intuition, or your higher self, talking to you. The more you lean into that knowledge, the higher your overall frequency or vibration will be. I know you might be hearing a lot of this for the first time, and I can sound kinda wacky. But trust me. Do the research yourself. These teachings have changed my life and made me enjoy being a nurse again.

I no longer hate going to work. I am still in pain after 20 years as a staff nurse: lifting people takes a toll on the body. But I can honestly feel love for being a nurse, and I know I am truly caring for my patients. I still get tired and cranky from time to time, but for the most part, I love being able to love on others.

Once we started spending time with Michelea, her husband Ed, and their team, our lives really started to improve. They were our upline in Amway and became our dearest friends. Once a week, we would all get together and celebrate each other's wins. The time we spent celebrating together helped improve our mental outlook each week.

We got to spend time with multimillionaires and learn how they made their lives better through reading and growing. I wanted to be a better person. I developed the motto to be *better than I was yesterday* and my only competition in this life is myself from the day before.

After four years of constantly improving my mindset and upleveling my self-care, I can no longer tolerate negative people. I was at work one day when a constantly miserable nurse was whining and complaining. My response to her was, "Ew gross. Your negativity is sticky! Take it somewhere else."

I am not sure she understood me, but all I knew was I could feel how gross her constant bitching was. I do not believe that people, especially nurses, understand how much their mindset affects their work. I started to do some research on the subject, and a lot of studies show how nurses who are unhappy actually perform poorly, making patient safety suffer. I used this research to complete my master's degree. I developed a resiliency program for new nurses. If I can impart one drop of wisdom to you, it is to manage your negativity.

Over the next few years, I dug deep into meditation and manifestation. I researched and integrated the practice into my life. I became a health coach from the Institute for Integrative Nutrition (IIN). I started my own health coaching business. I got certified in Reiki (energy healing) after experiencing some amazing healing effects from receiving reiki and learning about energy. We are made of energy. Our hearts literally conduct electricity. Let that soak in. This concept still messes with my head because if we are energy and energy cannot be created and cannot be destroyed, then we must just change forms. I have seen so many people cross over to another realm that I cannot turn away and say heaven and hell do not exist. How many nurses do you know who have stories of patients who have been what we call dead but come back and talked about it?

I can very vividly remember an older gentleman who appeared to us as *gone*. We were sternal rubbing him and got no response. I did the pen on the toe as hard as I could and got no response. He still had slow vitals though. We were getting ready to call a stroke alert because the physician was there and could not get the guy to respond to us. Then all of a sudden, he opened his eyes, *and he was pissed*. He yelled at us that he was with his wife, and how dare we bring him back. I can recall that moment as if I was standing right there. He kept telling everyone he was with his wife. She was holding his hand—mind you she had been dead for some time.

The more I research, and the more I dig into the world of manifestation, I realize that's what the successful people in life are doing. This knowledge is out there for everyone if you are willing to be open and learn to use the world of energy to your advantage. If you are willing to trust me and dig deep into your own mind, I promise the rewards of this work are amazing. I am living my purpose. My dream. I want to shout from the rooftops: *I love being a nurse!* I love being able to look into other human's eyes, and say, "I see you." I am able to tap into my intuition to help others. I believe the hippies from the '60s were right—we need more peace, love, and healing in this world. I stand as a beacon of light in the nursing world that you can heal your own wounds and still love being a nurse.

Some of you may not love nursing. Some of you may find that your true passion is something else, and that's OK. *Heal anyway.* Healing your own trauma is worth the pain. It is worth the hard work. It's worth all the tears shed for they are just watering the flowers of a beautiful life to bloom. The tears are seeds of kindness you get to plant. I know not everyone has pain or trauma to heal, and that is a beautiful story. I did and still do, and if you do, that is OK.

My goal is to tell my story and my truth so it may help a nurse who loves her profession but is worn down from taking on too much of everyone else's energy. I want to encourage others to learn, to heal, and to protect their own being so they can continue their career from a more centered and loving space.

Chapter 7
Shit Nursing School Didn't Teach You But Should Have

"If you have the ability to love, love yourself first."
~ Charles Bukowski

Though most of this book talks about my personal life, I also felt called to speak about some of the stressors I faced as a nurse. I have been an adjunct instructor for different nursing schools since I completed my master's degree in nursing education in 2021 and have seen how different nursing schools have become. When I was in my ADN program at CCAC, I was taught how to make a bed with hospital corners. My students didn't even know what those were. Hell, some programs do not even emphasize bathing the patients which was the only thing we were solely responsible for as student nurses. We were in the nursing homes for the first year learning how to actually care for people, feed them, and nurture them. Now, they are all about critical care and getting students as much experience off the unit as on the unit. Even now, there are still a lot of things that I feel are left out of the school programs. For example, they neglect to teach that the diseases you are learning about in school are often manifested because a person has emotions and feelings that get trapped in their tissues and fester, becoming the disease. Or like how somatic breathing techniques focus on the energy stuck in the body. Or how trauma at an early age sets people up for more disease in their bodies.

Those concepts would not only help nurses heal their patients but would also help the nurses heal themselves.

Humans are meant to feel emotions, but nurses are told to suck it up. With everything that we deal with day in and day out, though, it's nearly impossible to keep sucking it up year after year after year. You will explode! Whether it's with your patients or your family, it will definitely happen.

The problem is that we aren't taught how to cope. And we feel guilty, so it all piles on. It's not like you can tell your patient that you couldn't answer their call bell fast enough because you just spent the last 30 minutes doing CPR and pushing meds trying to save the life of the patient in the room next door. You walk out after the code is called and move on to the next patient. You don't get time to process the events. You are not afforded the time to reflect. It's all business. And people wonder why nurses become so cynical.

Instead of focusing on the new patient we just walked in to serve, sometimes we are stuck back in the last room. *What could I have done differently? What did I miss? Did I do everything I could for them? Could I have saved them? What if this and what if that?* You can destroy yourself with this thinking. But as a nurse, we all do it. As a nurse, you have to remind yourself you are still a human, and you will make mistakes, fail, learn, and grow.

To top it off, nurses are expected to not show emotions. Nurses are expected to handle everything professionally and not be human or have feelings. Heaven forbid if you show your feelings and cry; it makes you weak. When, in truth, it shows you are human. It is a strange profession we are in. We are here to care for others but we get the message, *don't show that you care too much* (shaking head in disgust). You can't get too attached to your patients because that is unprofessional also.

We see things that make other humans look at us like we should be placed on a psych hold if we talk about them. I saw a man with maggots crawling out of his nose after being found unresponsive in his car for who knows how long.

I got kicked in the chest by a girl pretending to be a psych patient when we were restraining her. I never go to the feet anymore. Lesson learned there. I bet my boobs are probably still hanging in the police office with a giant footprint in the center. (Yes, this is the incident I mentioned in the introduction.)

I got punched in the face for saving a young girl's life. Her friends dumped her off at the front entrance to the ER unconscious, so we threw her lifeless body on a stretcher and got her in a room while someone was getting the meds. I got the IV and slammed the Narcan in, and that bitch woke up swinging.

Like seriously, you were blue. Like, the color-in-the-crayon-box blue.

This is the thanks we get for saving your life: a fat lip. It's funny how I can see this scene playing out in my head, and I can remember what she looked like, but I have no idea what her name is. I do remember that we have matching tattoos. My ex-husband's friend was a local tattoo artist that used to give out free tattoos to girls. It was years later, that I realized it had the first initial of his name as part of the design of the tattoo.

I remember the first time I had to tell a family member that his loved one did not make it. Having to tell a young husband that his wife, age 36, was no longer of this earth still haunts me. I think about how they are doing. The kids are grown by now, but it still is as fresh in my mind as the day it happened. That was and still is a difficult conversation. No one told me how much I would learn to accept death. Being a nurse, you face your own mortality.

There are very few professions like ours. Nursing is evolving so fast, and there is so much pressure and responsibility, but we need to remember that we deserve to feel loved too.

I learned so many things over the years that I wish nursing school would have prepared me for, but I'm not sure I would have believed my teachers if they described some of the things I have experienced. Because we can deal with any number of crazy scenarios, I want to start you off with a few common things that nurses deal with in this chapter and give you some tools to handle them. It won't take away all the pain, anxiety, and apprehension, but it will help you shake loose of their hold.

Making a med error is super rare today because of all the technology to prevent it now in place, but it wasn't always like that. The thought of it happening causes us so much anxiety, and there is so much focus on preventing it, that it terrifies some nurses. What we should be doing is focusing on making it right and moving on to the next patient. A medication error is a big deal but schools should teach a nurse how to make a mistake, own it, and learn from it. *Everyone* makes mistakes. It's not a bad thing. Instead of panicking, maturely own your mistake and fill out an incident report. It's as simple as that.

The sad part is that school puts so much fear into students that if they make a tiny little mistake, they are going to get kicked out of nursing school. You are set up to feel fear from the first day. I think I still have PTSD from Mrs. Stevens's clinical. She terrified me. She made us write out all of our med cards to have for the day of clinical; then we were not allowed to look at them when passing meds—we had to have them memorized. She was horrified to see students looking those up on their phones during clinical. I have seen her in public a few times since school, and she was all, "Hey girl how are you? How's the kids?" like she was my best friend. I remember the one time at a Panera she came over and was all chatty and sweet. She walked away, and I looked at my daughter and told her how much that woman terrified me in nursing school. She laughed that even 15 years later this woman could still strike fear in me. I am sure everyone had that one teacher. I just do not understand using fear as a teaching technique.

One of the scenarios that leads to panic and fills nurses with anxiety is when you need to call the doctor at 3 a.m. Most hospitals now have a hospitalist who works overnight to cover these phone calls, but 20 years ago, we still had doctors who were private and not part of the hospitalist team. So, if something was wrong with their patient or if an order had been missed during that day and needed to be clarified, you had to call them. Most nurses have a story of their first call to the doctor. It's so funny to me now, but it wasn't as a new nurse. I was terrified to say the wrong thing or not know something if they asked me a question. But, now, I could give two shits about what the doctor thinks of me.

Nursing school should really address how to make the call to the doctor. If you're new, this sounds ridiculous, but stick with me. Imagine that it's night shift at like 3 a.m. when you realize the doctor never put the order in for medication, and now you are filled with anxiety because he is going to scream at you for waking him up for a "silly reason." The catch: you can't just put an order in without a doctor saying you can. That first call to clarify an order is so terrifying, especially when it's the doctor who hates being called and it's in the middle of the night.

I am sure you are shaking your head right now because you can feel the anxiety I am describing. I'm pretty sure we have all had this experience, especially as female nurses. After talking to so many male nurses, most of them do not have this experience. I do not fully understand why male nurses are treated with more respect from day one; they just are. It might stem from the days when nurses had to stand up and give the doctor their seat if they were all taken. It is so crazy to me that when I started, I was taught this concept. Just ask any nurse with 35 years or more of hospital nursing experience.

We also had to gather all the doctor's charts—because everything was still paper charting—and push the cart carrying all the patient's charts behind the doctor so he could do rounds. Heck when I first started nursing, we still had smoking rooms in the hospital. LIKE WHAT? Can you imagine?

Just crazy that this was all just 20 years ago. Yes, 20 years ago we did not have computer charting. Now we have to watch what we say in the room because most rooms are equipped with remote monitoring, and someone is always listening and reading our charts. It amazes me that technology has come so far, yet the profession is just as ass-backward as the day I started.

The first principle that should be covered in nursing school is self-care. Being taught from day one that you cannot pour from an empty cup would be more than helpful. I was taught that my patients come first, and, even in a fire, a nurse is never to save herself first, but to make sure all the patients are safe Then the nurse can get to safety. I remember my first real job as a nurse, (well second) but I only stayed at the VA for six months. I quit because I was a hormonal wreck—I was pregnant, but didn't know it, and everything annoyed me. Who knew pregnancy hormones could mess you up so much?

My first real job was a small community hospital that was short staffed—one of the biggest issues in most hospitals is that we are almost always short staffed. The nursing supervisor would say things like, "Are you really going to leave your unit short?" when you had a day off. I was young and naïve. I had no idea about the stereotype of the new nurse versus the experienced nurse and the old-ass nurse. Let me explain. The new nurse feels the guilt and will usually come in on her day off. The experienced nurse asks to switch a day so she still gets her time off. And the old-ass nurse? I answer the phone saying, "I started drinking with breakfast. Do you still want me drunk?" But it took me 20 years and the internet to learn this trick. I started as the new nurse who felt the guilt.

In the beginning, I felt so much guilt for taking a day off, but I also felt so much guilt for working so much and missing my children. It was a no-win situation for me, and I would fall for the guilt trip the nursing supervisors or the unit manager would give.

They would ask, (with an attitude) "Are you really going to take a day off?" or "Wouldn't you want someone to come in and help you when you are short staffed?"

Do you think they would ever take an assignment to help out? Hell no.

They walk around with their clipboard acting all important when we all know they can't take an assignment because most of them have been away from the bedside for so long they have no clue how to be a nurse anymore. Now, there are some good ones who do. There are always exceptions, but for the majority … you get the idea.

For years, I was guilted into always being at work, and I got so burned out. My marriage went to shit. Truthfully, it just highlighted how miserable the marriage already was, and it certainly put pressure on it.

I am grateful for this learning experience now because I can stand as the beacon to help prevent other nurses from caving to the guilt. As nurses, we give so much more of our energy to our work than most professions. We see people at their worst. We hold their hands as they are dying or close to it. We are the ones there when they get the bad news of a terminal diagnosis. We are the ones to see them at their weakest moment. Being in that space on a regular basis requires us to spend more time than other professions on our self-care.

Have you ever really thought about why you are so cranky after a shift? Or how about when you flip from days to nights and still try to be present for your family but feel like you are failing on all levels?

You might be experiencing burnout or compassion fatigue or whatever fancy term the big wigs or gurus want to call it right now. Honestly, our profession has been pushing nurses to take on more and more responsibility every year. We have finally hit a breaking point. The good thing that came from the COVID-19 pandemic was the wakeup call for management to realize that nurses need to be cared for too.

I have seen more wellness programs started for staff. At one facility, we actually have a wellness nurse who teaches meditation. At a recent staff meeting, we had a whole presentation on self-care. So, they are starting to see the importance of it … and that we need more than just a few pizzas. More money for putting up with no secretary or aides is nice, but as we care for the same amount of patients or even more, it's still not the answer.

Do nurses deserve more money? Absolutely! But that's not all. More money just helps the disrespect not feel so bad, but there is a point when the disrespect is so much that the money isn't even worth it. There comes a time in the level of burnout when you need to focus on making *you* happy to be able to keep being a nurse.

Think about these questions:

Are you always miserable at work? You might be feeling burned out!

Do you get chest pain or anxiety driving to work or getting ready for a shift? You might be feeling burned out!

Do you work so much extra that even the frequent flies with dementia remember you? You might be feeling burnout!

Do your children say things like, "Mom (or Dad) is in a bad mood again?" You might be feeling burnout!

So, now that you are thinking … if you realized that you are burned out from being a nurse (hint: you probably are if you've worked more than a month), here are some of the things that saved me and reinvigorated my nursing career.

Back in those early days, I used to always say, "I'm such a black cloud." "I always get the worst patients."

I had no idea about the Law of Attraction or manifesting my future. That sort of talk just kept me feeling stuck, awful, and hopeless. Be careful what you put out in the universe.

Now that I have spent the last 12 years learning and healing my burnout, I am here to hopefully help you have an easier or shorter time of healing to begin loving being a nurse again.

The first step is to realize that the symptoms you are feeling are normal.

Next, recognize that each of us brings our different backgrounds and our stories with us into our career. You can either learn to love your story and use it to help others, or you can let it eat at you till you become a bitter, old, bitchy nurse. Maybe you are already the old grouchy nurse on your unit. You know the one: everyone needs you but is afraid to ask you questions because you complain of everything you still need to do. No matter how good the nurse is, if someone is helping you, she is never doing it correctly. I'm cracking myself up because I admit that sometimes, *I'm the old cranky nurse*, and some days, I can be so much more helpful. It really depends on how much self-care I got to do that week.

During the weeks I do not get to do much self-care, I struggle. I am cranky and miserable. My husband unfortunately usually gets yelled at more when I am having a bad week, and I do not take time for myself. He is so supportive! I am truly blessed to have him in my life.

If I am really stressed out, my favorite self-care activity is going to put my feet in the creek and just listen to the water flow. Incidentally, the cover photo is of one of my favorite creeks. I know I am in a better mood when I start to feel more comfortable watching the water flow down the creek than when I stare upstream and in contrast watch the creek flow at me. When it is easy to watch the creek flow downstream, I know that my stress has traveled away with the water. When I am more comfortable watching the creek flow at me, and fighting against the current, I know, energetically, that I am not releasing something I should be.

When I started to learn about how each of us is energy and everything is energy, I was so caught up in the science of it all. So, I started looking into quantum physics and the theory of multiple universes. I still do not understand much of it, but I do understand the Law of Attraction and how the energy you put out in the world comes back to you. This is where I use the creek to help me gauge where my energy is flowing. I want to go with the flow of the universe and not fight it. I want my life to flow naturally as the creek does.

If it is a nice day, riding on the back of my husband's Harley is a good way to feed my soul. I grew up riding on the back of my dad's

Harley. It was always a safe space for me. Writing this book has given me so much confidence that I actually bought myself a Harley. So, we can either ride together or I can ride on the back. I also like to just sit in the woods. As a young girl, I would spend hours just sitting in the woods near our home. I would listen to the birds and the sounds of nature. I found out that trees actually absorb our negative energy and help us to release the anger and fear we have bottled up inside. So, sometimes, I will go hug a tree. These activities have all helped me cope with the day-to-day stress of being a nurse.

I am not sure what activity will help you to feel calm, but I hope you explore what makes you feel joy. I am sure there are so many more like quilting, sewing, or crocheting, even fishing, hunting, or going shooting. For some, it could be hiking or bicycling, maybe swimming or skiing; it could be reading or writing. There are thousands of activities people can do to relax. Some like to garden and some like to paint. What I hope to accomplish with this book is to inspire you, as a nurse, to do something for yourself other than sleep on your days off. Or just do the things that need done like clean the carpets. I want to inspire you to dig deep into something that brings you pure joy, so the next time a family member of a patient tells you how awful you are, you can picture one of these things that you did to bring you joy.

The moral of this story is that you were designed to feel loved. You deserve love. Do not ever let a job make you feel otherwise because being a nurse is the most amazing career you could have chosen. You devoted your life to caring for others and that deserves *so much honor*, so tell your boss to shut up. Wait, don't really do that. You might get fired. But fuck that. You're a nurse; you can get a job anywhere. We always need nurses.

Putting yourself first is not an act of selfishness; it is an act of love. It will make you a better parent and a better partner. Having a self-care routine that fills your soul and makes your cup overflow will make you a better nurse and a better human. Every person on this planet deserves to feel loved.

Putting yourself first is not selfish.

Being selfish is only worrying about *me, me, me*.

As a nurse, it's hard to be selfish when your entire career is thinking about other people.

There are major differences between self-care and being selfish, so do not let anyone ever make you feel like you are being selfish when you are doing things that feed your soul.

Most people do not understand the mental energy it takes to care for others.

As nurses, we choose to love on strangers as a career, but that doesn't mean we have to put ourselves last either.

Go out, and do something that brings you joy. Take your days off. Love yourself so you can love others. And thank you for being a nurse.

Conclusion

"Courage is to never let your actions be influenced by your fears."[10]
~ Arthur Koestler

I want to leave you in a better place than where I found you. In the words of Jim Rohn, "You aren't a tree."[11] Meaning, if you do not like where you are, then move. You can change. You can grow. You can better yourself. You do not have to keep dealing with the same bullshit year after year. I look at some nurses and wonder how they still get up in the morning because they have been doing the same thing over and over and are so afraid of change that they are stuck. You are a nurse. You are never stuck. You are always needed. You can always change. I hope if you have learned only one thing from my story it is that *change is a good thing*.

I always strive to learn something new every day, even if it's a small tidbit of random knowledge. I just want to keep my mind growing.

I hope you now have a good self-care routine and think about what makes you feel happy. I want every nurse to love being a nurse, and if you do not love it, then find something that you do love. Not everyone who goes to nursing school becomes a nurse but every nurse goes to nursing school. There are a lot of people in this world who started nursing school and either failed out or quit when things got hard. You did not. You fought hard to get the degree and practice as a nurse. You endured the stress and the hardships of forgoing family functions for the years of school

---

[10] https://quotefancy.com/quote/758493/Arthur-Koestler-Courage-is-never-to-let-your-actions-be-influenced-by-your-fears

[11] https://www.youtube.com/watch?v=L7MuAX-6Yzg

because nursing school is a full time job that you don't get paid for. Being a nurse needs to be celebrated more than just one week a year—that now we have to share with teachers, I might add. I may be a little jaded, since we have that week because Florence Nightingale's birthday is on May 12th. Teachers, I love you, but you should pick a different week. But I digress.

I hope I have imparted enough of my growing pains from over the years that you feel empowered that you, too, can overcome any obstacle. I have been through some shit in my life, but I would not change any of it; it has made me who I am today.

As a trauma survivor, it was always so hard to enjoy the good times. I kept waiting for the preverbal other shoe to drop. You know, I was expecting the next bad thing to happen. I had to spend years retraining my brain to expect the good things. I remember reading the book *Hardwiring your Brain for Happiness* by Rick Hanson. The author goes into great detail about how the brain works and how it is fundamental that our brains try to protect us from bad stuff. Way back in human history, the brain had to sense danger and protect us from predators.

Today, we don't have too many predators, depending on where you live, but we do still have an ego that likes to keep us small and safe. I named mine Sammy. I named her so I could talk to her. At first, it was hard, and I felt weird. But now, when things get scary, I look in the mirror and talk to her. She is just a part of my personality, and we have learned to work together. I know this sounds a little strange, but this is the technique I learned to use so I did not let fear hold me back. I let her talk me out of writing this book for almost ten years. I always knew I wanted to be a writer. I just never pulled the trigger until now. So when I start to feel fear, I picture me handing Sammy some crystals and telling her to go play in the backseat. I am driving this bus, and we are doing whatever it is I am afraid of because I have learned that freedom is on the other side of fear.

One example of a fear I knew I wanted to overcome was that I kept being afraid to ride with my husband on his motorcycle at night. I would go for a ride, but we always had to be back before dark, until one night, when we went on a memorial ride for a good friend that was two hours away. We were riding home at sunset, and it was absolutely gorgeous. Because I faced that fear and did it anyway, the confidence I gained was tremendous. That was three years ago. I keep doing little things I am afraid of, and my confidence is growing.

As a new nurse, I have been treated so badly by the older nurses, pretty much tortured. I was made fun of and criticized for everything. There was one nurse who was so scary to me. She was never happy, no matter what. I could spend the last two hours of my shift making my room perfect and my charting perfect, and she would find something to bitch at me for. She was the type of nurse who refused to let anyone help her with anything, and you did not dare go into her room if her pump was beeping. She would chew you out.

Well, funny thing is, she actually pushed me to get my CCRN, which is the critical care nurse certification. I was determined to prove to her that I was a good nurse. I got it, and she couldn't have cared less. I got my BSN, and she didn't care. She still made me tremble every time I had to give her a report. It turns out, she ended up being my patient one day with an abscessed tooth that made her septic because, as the typical nurse does, she ignored it. Even *that* did not change her mind. I don't know what happened to her after I left that job, but I ran into her like three years later at a different job where we ended up working together. She asked me if we could talk. She ended up apologizing to me, and we have been friends since and still talk and go to lunch. It's funny how, back then, I was so intimidated by a nurse like that. Now, ha, I could give two shits if anyone at work likes me. Seriously. It's nice to get along with your coworkers, but as a nurse, you realize there are just some bitches you can't please.

And, I am not for everyone, but I'm OK with that. I have developed a new sense of self-confidence, so no matter what, no one's opinion of me is going to make my heart stop beating or my lungs stop breathing. Haters gonna hate. Honestly, if hate is directed at me, it's usually because I represent something for them that they are not ready to handle. Maybe a past hurt or a trauma … or they are just plain mean. I just say a prayer for that person and move on. If I am still working with the person, I will always help out another nurse no matter what. If they say they do not need help I say *OK* and walk away, but I will always offer.

I would love to be able to positively impact every nurse, but I am just kind to everyone and offer to help. I'm a utility nurse. I will help lift a patient, clean an ass, and feed them. I will look at your kids', dog's, or cat's pictures. Hell, I will even help you pick your next husband or listen while you rant about your wife. I have learned that most of us just need a friend or a helping hand. I never want a nurse to feel how alone I have felt.

It definitely changes you when you feel like no one in the world would miss you if you died. Reach out to me if you feel all alone. I have a huge list of people I support and am a cheerleader for. We may have never met in person, but I root for them and give them encouragement. I have been to the depths of despair, as you have read, and I want to be the love this world needs. I spend my time now trying to show strangers love and kindness. I try to offer compliments to strangers because you never know if that's what they need to change their lives. I hope that reading my story has given you a sense of community in the nursing world that lets you know you are not alone, that someone else has experienced similar things, and not just survived but is thriving. This world has enough hate. Be the light. Be a lighthouse nurse.

If you feel you need more, I am available for one-on-one coaching. I *help nurses love nursing while healing themselves.* Check out my website and book a session.

Website: LoriLewicki.com

Nursing Terms

Bridle: the device used to secure the ng tube

C-Diff: a germ that disrupts normal flora of the gut when taking antibiotics and can become a huge infection causing liquid projectile stool

MSN: master's degree in nursing

NCLEX: the national testing board for licensing (national council licensure examination)

NG tube: a nasal gastric tube that stays in the stomach and is inserted through the nose

Resection: removal of part of your intestines followed by reconnection to a different section, removing the diseased part. A very common bowel surgery for Crohn's patients. A colostomy bag is not needed.

Sternal rub: grinding your knuckles into a person's sternum to check for consciousness, usually when they are not breathing and not responding

Resources

Suicide help: call or text 988 in the United States, https://988lifeline.org/

Addiction Recovery Centers of America: 1-800-RECOVERY, https://recoverycentersofamerica.com/

Gambling addiction: 1-800-GAMBLER, https://www.ncpgambling.org/

Alcoholics Anonymous: https://www.aa.org/ (has meetings in every state)

Celebrate Recovery: https://celebraterecovery.com/ (has meetings in most states) A faith-based program helping people overcome hurts, pains, bad habits, etc.

National Institutes of Mental Health: https://www.nimh.nih.gov/

National Alliance on Mental Health: https://www.nami.org/

* You can always ask your family doctor for referrals to mental health professionals

Books I Read to Improve Myself

The 4-Hour Work Week by Tim Ferriss

The 7 Habits of Highly Effective People by Stephen R. Covey

Chakra Healing: A Beginner's Guide to Self-Healing Techniques that Balance the Chakras by Margarita Alcantara

Change Your Brain, Change Your Body: Use Your Brain to Get and Keep the Body You Have Always Wanted by Daniel G. Amen, MD

The Compound Effect: Jumpstart Your Income, Your Life, Your Success by Darren Hardy

Don't Sweat the Small Stuff … and It's All Small Stuff: Simple Ways to Keep the Little Things from Taking Over Your Life by Richard Carlson

Emotional Intelligence: Why It Can Matter More Than IQ by Daniel Goleman

The Five Love Languages by Gary Chapman

The Five Love Languages: The Secret to Love That Lasts by Gary Chapman

The Five Second Rule by Mel Robbins

Go for No! Yes is the Destination, No is How You Get There by Richard Fenton and Andrea Waltz

Grit: The Power of Passion and Perseverance by Angela Duckworth

Hardwiring Happiness: The New Brain Science of Contentment, Calm, and Confidence by Rick Hanson

How to be a People Magnet: Finding Friends and Lovers and Keeping them for Life by Leil Lowndes

How to Have your Best Year Ever by Jim Rohn

How to Talk to Anyone: 92 Little Tricks for Big Success in Relationships by Leil Lowndes

I Hate You—Don't Leave Me: Understanding the Borderline Personality by Jerold Kreisman, MD, and Hal Straus

Limitless Expanded Edition: Upgrade Your Brain, Learn Anything Faster, and Unlock Your Exceptional Life by Jim Kwik

The Master Key System by Charles F. Haanel

Mind Hacking: How to Change Your Mind for Good in 21 Days by Sir John Hargrave

Mind over Medicine: Scientific Proof that you Can Heal Yourself by Lissa Rankin, MD

Mindset: The New Psychology of Success by Carol Dweck

Revolutionary Productivity by Katie Mazzocco

The Science of Likability by Patrick King

The Secret by Rhonda Byrne

Stop Walking on Eggshells: Taking Your Life Back When Someone You Care About Has Borderline Personality Disorder by Paul Mason, MS, and Randi Kreger

Thank & Grow Rich: A 30-Day Experiment in Shameless Gratitude and Unabashed Joy by Pam Grout

Think and Grow Rich by Napoleon Hill

The Traveler's Gift: Seven Decisions that Determine Personal Success by Andy Andrews

You are a Badass: How to Stop Doubting your Greatness and Start Living an Awesome Life by Jen Sincero

You are the Team: 6 Simple Ways Teammates Can Go From Good To Great by Michael G. Rogers

About the Author

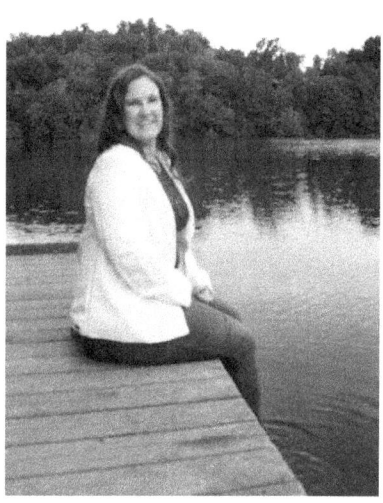

Lori Ann Lewicki is an ICU travel nurse, life and health coach for nurses, mother of four (ages 26, 24, 19 and 3) and caregiver to her elderly father—so she never gets a day off from being a nurse. She is also an advocate for living your dreams.

Writing *Surviving Shit Creek* empowered Lori to follow her own dreams. Because she has grown so much as a nurse and a human, she hopes to inspire others to go after their dreams and never quit learning to be better than the day before.

Lori graduated from Community College of Allegheny County with her ADN in nursing in 2004 and, being a nerd, also graduated with an associate's degree in psychology. She obtained her BSN in 2006 from California University of Penn., her PHRN in 2010, had her first CCRN from 2007-2010, her MSN in 2022, and retested for her CCRN in 2024. Lori has also been a certified health coach since 2019. She has worked in the ICU, in the ER, on the ambulance, in medical review, in home care, and as a nursing instructor over her career.

One of Lori's dreams was to buy a Harley and get her motorcycle license, which she did in celebration of the completion of *Surviving Shit Creek*.

www.ingramcontent.com/pod-product-compliance
Lightning Source LLC
Chambersburg PA
CBHW071204120626
46546CB00006B/2406